Mad Diet

How Your Diet Can Help You to Lose Weight and Cure Depression

Suzanne Lockhart

CORONET

This edition published in Great Britain in 2017 by Coronet
An imprint of Hodder & Stoughton
An Hachette UK company

First published in 2016

6

A CIP catalogue record for this title is available from the British Library

Paperback ISBN: 978 1 473 65706 9
Ebook ISBN: 978 1 473 65707 6

Printed and bound in Great Britain by Clays Ltd, Elcograf S.p.A.

Hodder & Stoughton policy is to use papers that are natural, renewable
and recyclable products and made from wood grown in sustainable
forests. The logging and manufacturing processes are expected to
conform to the environmental regulations of the country of origin.

Hodder & Stoughton Ltd
Carmelite House
50 Victoria Embankment
London EC4Y 0DZ

www.hodder.co.uk

Dedicated to all the amazing Glasgow grannies, especially mine – Elizabeth Lockhart. I love and miss you.

Contents

Acknowledgements

'Alone we can do so little, together we can do so much.'

– Helen Keller

With the wise words of Helen Keller in mind there are a few people I must acknowledge in the creation of this book, as without the love and support from each and every one of them *Mad Diet* wouldn't have made it from my head to the page.

Firstly, I would like to thank Veronica for encouraging me to join the food industry all those years ago, an experience which has changed my life for ever.

I must also thank my family for teaching me how to stand on my own two feet – an invaluable life lesson. You taught me never to give up, even when the chips were sometimes stacked against me.

A deep bow to Lorna, one of the most enlightened souls I've met on my journey and the lady who graciously taught me reiki and how to love myself again.

Grateful thanks to Jan, my guiding light over the years, whose insights helped to keep my compass pointing north when writing this book.

Special thanks to Karen McCreadie, who simplified my cumbersome prose and garbled research notes and transformed them into something worth reading. Without your input, *Mad Diet* would not be what it is and for that I am eternally grateful.

I'm also honoured at Irene McCabe's generosity in writing the foreword to *Mad Diet*. You are a talented and genuine healthcare professional that I am proud to call my friend.

And to my darling son, thank you for giving me the strength to keep going during those dark days. You saved me from myself and continue to teach me every day. I love you more than you will ever know.

'A misty morning may become a clear day.'

– Scottish proverb

Foreword for Mad Diet

Melancholia shows no mercy. If you currently suffer from depression or care about someone who does, or you just have to look at a doughnut and you gain weight, then this book is for you.

Every so often a book comes along which changes the game and *Mad Diet* is definitely a game changer. This is not just another diet book. It joins the dots on what is *really* going on with our food and medicine and is likely to connect with your intuition, an 'inner knowing' that goes far deeper than words. It is also a call to action, encouraging Western women to take their power back and make the transition to a healthier, happier life.

The intention of the author shouts even louder than the words on the page. Her message has integrity as it comes from two different, yet powerful, sources. First, the book is a product of her own personal experiences suffering from depression and weight problems, and second it is the product of years of research and her professional insights into the real causes of physical and mental illness. Mental health, food science and nutrition are serious subjects that have been covered by many academics, scientists, researchers and authors but rarely does the life-changing information reach the people those authors are actually writing about – those who so desperately need it. Occasionally a book emerges that can change that and resonate with the people that are actually living the nightmare. I believe *Mad Diet* is that book!

There is something about Suzanne Lockhart's writing that is instantly likeable. She describes her west of Scotland, working-class upbringing in a way that will invoke many childhood memories for those of us who grew up in the 1960s, 1970s and 1980s. Lockhart has taken on huge topics – food, medicine, agriculture and industry – and distilled the scope of work into a book which is easily understood and clearly explains why so many women (and men) are struggling with weight and mental health problems. The reader is also encouraged to do their own research while using the information in the book as an easy step guide to self-healing.

Some information regarding the food industry may come as a revelation to you. It was to me, and has left me wondering how we have come to a place where profit appears to be more important than people, their health or the planet. Many of us take for granted and trust that the food available to us is nutritionally beneficial but it is clear that this may not be the case. Suzanne has researched the work of many eminent scientists and doctors who have inspired her to bring forth this knowledge.

I have been an independent nutritional researcher for over 30 years and as a newspaper columnist based in Scotland I fully understand the health challenges facing women in the UK. I also understand the importance of natural healthcare and the growing need for us to take more responsibility for our own health.

This book really grabbed my attention. Not only does it bring together the old clichés of how 'our psychology becomes our biology' and 'we are what we eat', but goes far deeper to explain in easy-to-understand terms how the food we eat affects both our physical and mental health and how making conscious decisions about what we put in our shopping trolleys can radically change our lives.

Everyone gets the blues from time to time, but depression is a vile condition that rarely comes with much sympathy. Unlike many physical conditions, mental torment is usually invisible and as such is too often ignored or dismissed by society. It often lies hidden, anonymous, undetected, to those looking in as the sufferer puts on the face of the sad clown. Having suffered from a short spell of hormonally related depression and postnatal depression in my twenties I too speak from experience. I wish

I had had this information to hand in those dark days, when even as a nutritional researcher I did not have the energy, joie de vivre, nor the concentration to look for a way out of the darkness. Thankfully, I stumbled upon magnesium and vitamin B complex which together with a change in diet helped immensely and I have never looked back. Others have not been so lucky.

I have tested the teachings in *Mad Diet* to great effect. The power and simplicity of this book could be life-changing but please don't take my word for it. Why not find out for yourself and try it.

And when it works, when you finally feel better than you've felt in years – spread the word.

Irene McCabe is an independent nutritional researcher and health writer, Scottish newspaper columnist and complementary medicine practitioner.

Introduction: Reality Check

'Tell me what you eat, and I'll tell you what you are.'

– Anthelme Brillat-Savarin

So, you've just bought a book called *Mad Diet* which means I can probably make a few reasonably accurate assumptions about you. Most likely you saw the word 'diet' and a frisson of hope flashed across your mind. Maybe this one is going to be the one that makes the difference. Whether you're carrying a few extra pounds or are really struggling with some serious weight issues you probably don't like what you see in the mirror any more. Most of us know what that feels like – at least anyone who's ever bought a diet book does! The clothes shopping for a new suit or summer dress for an upcoming wedding – those awful four-way mirrors under spotlights that allow you to see the unwelcome expanding contours in all their high beam, widescreen glory. Chances are you've got a dozen or more diet books in your house (probably stuffed under the bed or boxed ready for the next charity shop donation run). Come on, admit it – you've tried everything from the cabbage soup diet (windy side effects made this one particularly challenging if you worked in close proximity to other people) to the grapefruit diet, the Atkins diet to the South Beach diet and beyond. It's likely that a few of these approaches even worked for a while, but they also probably made you miserable so eventually you 'fell off the wagon' and put the weight back on. Usually, with a little bit extra just to remind you that you'd failed. And this endless cycle certainly doesn't help your state of mind. Hence the 'mad' part of the title – perhaps you, like millions of women around the world, are struggling with mental health issues. 'Mental health

14

issues' is a pretty 'heavy' term but actually mental health can range from irritability and trouble sleeping, to anxiety or full-blown panic attacks, through to diagnosable challenges such as depression and bipolar disorder.

So if you're fat, mad or both – don't go anywhere, turn off your phone and bolt the door – this book is for you. But, before we begin I want to make a few things crystal clear – I've been called both – 'fat' and 'mad'. I don't look like a supermodel, I enjoy my fizzy plonk and I don't follow some impossibly difficult or expensive diet, but I am incredibly healthy and I've successfully overcome chronic mental health problems by following the steps I'll share with you in this book.

I'm an average woman who started life in a council estate in a working-class area of Glasgow in Scotland. Beyond the stereotypes of haggis eating, whisky drinking and kilt wearing, Scots are generally warm, funny and pretty blunt. We call a spade a spade and political correctness is often lost on us – so expect some straight-shooting in this book. If you're fat – own it, accept it and change it. If you're mad – own it, accept it and change it. I promise you it's possible and it won't require you to find countless extra hours a week, turn into Mary Berry or Julia Child overnight or find a hidden stash of cash – anyone can follow the advice in these pages to help wean themselves off antidepressants, lose weight, and maybe even look and feel ten years younger!

Something is Wrong

So why are so many of us fat, mad or both? Something is clearly very wrong.

And the really crazy thing is we all know it. We may not know what the problem is but instinctively we know something isn't quite what it should be.

I don't know about you, but when I was a child I didn't even know a vegetarian, never mind someone who was lactose intolerant or allergic to soy. There were no kids in my class at school who carried an EpiPen (adrenaline-injecting device) in case they had a close encounter with a peanut. Today you would be hard pressed to find a classroom in the UK or US that didn't have at least one child who was allergic to peanuts. In 2014 a four-year-old girl went into anaphylactic shock on a flight after a passenger ignored repeated warnings that the girl had a severe nut allergy and opened a packet of mixed nuts. To be clear, he wasn't sitting next to her, she didn't eat, touch or even see the nuts, and yet it was enough to almost kill her.

But it's not just peanuts, a growing number of people, especially children, are allergic to milk, eggs, wheat, soy, fish and shellfish to name just a few. In the UK each year the number of allergy sufferers increases by 5 per cent. Between 1992 and 2012 there was a 615 per cent increase in hospital admissions because of food allergies and the number of people suffering from food allergies in the UK has doubled in the last decade. In Europe it's estimated that 150 million people have allergies. In the US 55 per cent of the population test positive for one or more allergen. We now have conditions, diseases and disorders that didn't even exist in our grandparents' day – Crohn's, lupus, IBS, ME – the list is almost endless. In the US there are just under six million children diagnosed with ADHD and in the UK 130,000 children are diagnosed with severe ADHD. These are all relatively new health challenges that are not only costing us billions every year and putting enormous strain on healthcare but they are having a significant impact on our quality of life.

It never ceases to amaze me just how little regard we have for what we eat and drink. We are intelligent human beings, capable of space travel and mind-boggling innovation and invention, and yet we serve junk food in hospitals and consume food laden with ingredients we can't even pronounce and wonder why we don't feel like Usain Bolt. And while it may be obvious that we are not eating the right things if we are overweight – so far the link between what we consume and mental health has been completely ignored in the mainstream media. This book is going to set the record straight so you can get the information you need to make better choices, not only for your waistline but for your mental health too.

Our diet has changed, the way our food is produced, processed and even packaged has changed and these changes are having a profound impact on our physical and mental well-being. But it's taken me several decades to understand why.

In the 1980s having a chemical imbalance in your brain was barely understood by doctors and even less so by the average person on the street. Most people knew who shot J. R. Ewing in popular US soap opera *Dallas* but no one had heard of serotonin. Back then, when you got labelled with depression it was assumed that you had suffered some horrific childhood trauma or it just 'ran in the family'. At the time, I didn't know what was wrong but I knew something wasn't right so, like most of us, I went to my GP. I explained how I felt and within three minutes he handed me a prescription for antidepressants adding, 'Here, take these and don't worry, half your colleagues will be on them.'

I was never asked about my diet, no tests were run on the condition of my blood to establish if I had any nutrient deficiencies and I certainly wasn't asked about my life or the environment I was living in. Instead I was bundled out the door with a prescription for some pills and an appointment card to see a psychiatrist. The following years were a blur of monthly prescriptions, scab-picking sessions at the shrink's office and regular trips to the slimming club. By my thirties I was a whopping 224 pounds – which would be fine if I was six foot five inches tall. Unfortunately I am the same height as Kylie Minogue or Reese Witherspoon and I was almost as wide as I was tall. Plus, I was bloody miserable – every day was a battle.

Being depressed was one thing but dealing with obesity exhausted what little self-esteem I had left. The low-fat eating plans, gym memberships and – I'm ashamed to admit – illicit diet pills led me down a path of yo-yo dieting which just made my mental health issues worse. To be honest, I grappled with episodic notions of self-loathing, hopelessness and suicide.

Thankfully I managed to maintain my career during those dark years. Granted, I needed to lean on the occasional imaginary sick relative when the black dog held me captive in bed but like so many of us, I muddled through. And ironically my career became my salvation because I worked in the food industry. Through my work I became increasingly aware of the dangers lurking in our weekly shopping trolley and the potential link between cost-saving initiatives, increased use of additives and mental health problems, obesity and countless other modern-day conditions that simply did not exist 50 years ago. Working across 12 countries with various Fortune 500 food manufacturers, grocery retailers, farming groups and government organisations provided me with unique insight into the way in which our food is farmed, processed and marketed in the UK, Europe and North America.

As I was cutting my teeth in the industry developing new products and helping to create big brands in various food categories including bakery products, fresh produce, meat, confectionery and desserts, I quickly learned that the need to make a profit was vastly more important than the need to create nutritious or even safe food. Competition for supermarket shelf space meant that even the most honourable product developers, who initially took great pride in creating safe and healthy food for their customers, were being forced to find cost savings. Besides, if the Food and Drug Administration (FDA), United States Department of Agriculture (USDA), Department for Environment, Food and Rural Affairs (DEFRA), Food Standards Agency (FSA) and Canadian Food Inspection Agency (CFIA) approved a substance safe to eat, or a supply chain fit for purpose, nobody questioned the science behind such decisions or the morality of using synthetic or potentially unhealthy ingredients. If the government says it's OK, then it's OK – right?

Only it isn't OK. I still vividly remember countless sleepless nights after I was instructed to remove 20 per cent cost from a popular children's sausage brand. I lay there in the darkness, watching my bedside clock pass each hour. Twenty per cent cost saving meant 'remove the meat' – and at the very least it meant reduce the quality of the meat and add bulking agents and chemical flavour enhancers. I knew mothers who bought that product for their children. How was I going to look them in the eye knowing the true content of the product? Not long after I left that role and jumped over the fence to help track and measure the quality of our food up and down the supply chain but frankly it's an endless battle.

The 'behind the scenes' access to the food industry together with my own personal health problems ignited a passion to first heal myself and then use what I discovered to liberate millions of overweight, depressed woman from the living hell caused by crap food and addiction to antidepressants.

What we are eating is making us fat, mad and ill. And I'm not just talking about the obvious culprits like too much fat, sugar or processed foods. I'm talking about the hidden ingredients in so much of the food we consume and the production techniques that increase quantity but reduce nutritional quality. I'm talking about the loss of essential micronutrients from our food chain that are having a *profound* effect on global health and mental well-being.

We need to shout from the rooftops so that women everywhere understand that the government decisions to endorse certain food groups and products are often the result of corporate lobbying on the behalf of big business, not stringent testing and approval because they are safe and healthy. Even today, in the US for example, millions of dollars are being spent by big food manufacturers to prevent genetically modified (GM) labelling and to avoid country of origin labelling because the major food processors don't want to admit what is in the food they create or where it's produced. They know that knowledge will impact sales but we absolutely need that knowledge if we are to make good buying choices for ourselves and our families. Without proper labelling the small traditional farmers who care about what they produce are all at a profound disadvantage to the corporate giants who only care about profit and shareholder return. Plus, many of the worse culprits are cheaper processed, synthetic products masquerading as 'real food'. And frankly the people making the laws and passing these products fit for public consumption will *never* eat them and they certainly won't serve them to their children. Did you know, for example, that the food served in the Houses of Parliament is all GM-free – there isn't a genetically modified ingredient within half a mile of Westminster! Suffice to say politicians and food policymakers are not eating frozen horsemeat burgers and children's sausages stuffed with 'E'-numbers and 'meat' you wouldn't give your dog. But busy mums and lower-income families are and it's making them sick, sick, sick.

Part One of this book will be dedicated to defining the problem so we are really clear about just what we are up against. Part Two will then explore the history of the problem so that you can appreciate what happened to bring us to this point. You may not think this is important and may be more interested in getting to the solution so you can start to take some action and feel better. But, change is not always easy – even when we desperately need to change and want to change. Knowing how we got here and all the behind the scenes wheeling and dealing will hopefully fuel your anger and keep you motivated towards your goal of better health. We'll also look at the history of medicine and how many doctors are as ignorant of the facts as we are. Part Three is the 'get educated' section, where we will look at the influence of marketing on our buying choices and how we are being manipulated and hoodwinked, and what we can do about it. It's only fair to warn you that I do mention various biological systems and you may come across medical or technical words and phrases that are unfamiliar, even if you can still remember some high school biology. Please don't be put off by this. I've deliberately kept this to an absolute minimum because, let's be honest, it can be excruciatingly boring to read, but some explanation is often necessary to ensure you take this information seriously and don't simply dismiss it as my *opinion*.

Everything I say in this book is verifiable and a snapshot of the science demonstrating it is listed, by chapter, in the reference section. And finally, Part Four details the action plan which looks at all the food groups and what we need to know for each one, how to be a savvy 'mood food' shopper and how to successfully supplement your diet to ensure we get the right micronutrients for optimal physical and mental well-being. This section will also give you a programme for how best to safely wean yourself off antidepressants if you are currently on them. These drugs should never be stopped cold turkey – instead you need to take the dose down slowly with the support of your GP, once you have made some positive changes to your diet.

I am eternally grateful for my experience in the food industry because it gave me a unique insight into the obscured machinations of our food supply and allowed me to finally connect the dots between what we are putting in our shopping trolleys and our rapidly declining physical and mental health. This book is going to explain why, and most importantly how, you can heal yourself.

Part One
Defining the Problem

'If people let the government decide what foods they eat and what medicines they take, their bodies will soon be in as sorry a state as the souls who live under tyranny.'

– Thomas Jefferson

Chapter 1: Mad Fat Epidemic

'Any food that requires enhancing by the use of chemical substances should in no way be considered a food.'

– John H. Tobe

Ironically, although it has taken me decades to accumulate the knowledge, experience and information that has allowed me to connect the dots between what we consume and our physical and mental health, my granny knew the truth long before I did.

I adored my granny and I would see her regularly throughout my young life. She was a typical strong, no-nonsense Glaswegian woman who lived in Possilpark. At the time Possilpark was not just one of the poorest places in Glasgow but the whole of the UK. It was, however, also a thriving working-class community built around the Clyde steel industry. It was the women who held the community together, especially after the First World War. If the husbands and sons did return from the war they were understandably changed by their experiences. And in those days there was no counselling or appreciation of post-traumatic stress disorder (PTSD) and there were certainly no support groups. Before the NHS was created in 1947 everyone had to pay to go to the doctor so women like my granny just didn't go. They couldn't afford it. Instead they focused on how to keep the doctor at bay with a few inexpensive supplements. I still remember standing in the kitchen each morning to receive one teaspoon of cod liver oil and if I had an upset tummy I'd also get one teaspoon of Milk of Magnesia. I couldn't decide which was worse – the fish oil that I'd burp back up throughout the day or the unpleasant chalky texture to the Milk of Magnesia. But we had it every morning without fail – old-school preventative medicine Glasgow-style.

The medicine cabinet in my granny's house contained:

- Milk of Magnesia (magnesium)
- Andrews liver salts (bicarbonate of soda and magnesium)
- Cod liver oil (omega-3, vitamins A and D)
- Bronchial cough mixture (active ingredients – aniseed, capsicums, ginger, cloves)
- Zinc
- Castor oil
- Aspirin
- Epsom salts (poured into the bath the magnesium would be absorbed through the skin)

That was the medicine taken care of. As for the food – there was always a pan of home-made soup on the range and everything was made from scratch.

Life was tough. Granny would cook with the fruit and vegetables my granddad had grown in the allotment or what was available locally. She made her own bread and the meat would often come from the local farmer. Every year a few families in the neighbourhood would club together and buy a whole cow, butcher it themselves and distribute the meat between the families. But these were not lifestyle choices – they came down to necessity.

They didn't have a lot of money but they were incredibly healthy and both my grandparents lived until they were well into their eighties – despite my granddad's 40- 60-a-day Capstan full-strength cigarette habit and his penchant for whisky.

Granny died when I was in my early teens. I still remember the grief and the huge hole she left in my life. But it took me years to realise that my regular intake of Milk of Magnesia, cod liver oil and home-made food had kept me healthy. Without it, my physical and mental health soon started to decline. As I deteriorated, I put it down to being a teenager, exam stress and strained relationships with other family members. What I now realise is that the micronutrients in my granny's preventative medicine routine and her wholesome, nutrient-rich home cooking was what saved me from the mental and physical health issues that were to become part of my daily life. And I was not alone…

Today we are slap bang in the middle of the 'mad fat epidemic'. One in four Western women is taking antidepressants. In Europe 38 per cent of people have a diagnosable mental illness. And one in three Western women are obese despite government healthy eating guidelines and a plethora of diet books published each year teaching us how to lose weight and stay healthy – many of which you and I probably own.

Population data now shows that obesity rates and diagnosis of mental illness began rising in the mid-1980s and have been rising steadily ever since. So what the hell happened in the 80s?

Food Production Started to Change

Changes to food production following the Second World War were really having an impact by the 1980s. Small, family-owned, traditionally run farms made way for industrial farming (whether they wanted to or not). It's worth pointing out here that when it comes to farming, the 'good guys' are the remaining small, traditionally run, often family-owned farms that put quality and animal welfare above quantity. If you still have some 'good guys' in your community support them, otherwise all we'll have left are the 'bad guys'. The 'bad guys' are the large-scale commercial farms, often owned by conglomerates where quantity is king – regardless of the quality or animal welfare.

An over-reliance on pesticides and engineered animal feed used by the 'bad guys' started to alter the body fat composition and chemistry of these mass-produced animals. Chicken, by far the most popular meat in the Western diet, is now produced twice as fast as it was 30 years ago. This is achieved by feeding chickens a high-fat diet but high fat in means high fat out. As a result the fat content in chicken, ironically often assumed to be a low-fat alternative to red meat, has increased from 2 per cent to 22 per cent in just 30 years. This has also altered the balance of vital fatty acids in chicken, which means you are almost certainly eating too much omega-6 and not enough omega-3 – especially if chicken is a large part of your diet. The right balance of omega-3 to omega-6 is essential for optimum brain function and the ratio should be 1:3 but people eating a Western diet now consume around 1:16, leading to inflammation and mental dysfunction. Again my granny didn't eat mass-produced chicken that arrived in plastic trays from the supermarket. My granddad would get his chicken from the local farmer. This imbalance in fatty acids doesn't occur when chickens are raised naturally (or organically) on a diet of plant matter, insects and other small bugs and grubs. In those days the farmer's chickens were let out of their 'hen house' in the morning and would spend the day scratching through the farmyard and hedgerows, happily laying their eggs with bright yellow yolks.

Mass production has also depleted the nutrient content of crops. If land is used over and over again to grow the same crop without crop rotation or giving the land a rest then there are fewer minerals in the soil, which means there are fewer nutrients in industrially farmed cereals, fruits and vegetables. If the nutrients are not in the soil, they won't be in the plants that are grown in the soil and we won't get the nutrients when we eat those plants. To facilitate this endless growing cycle the land is usually treated with chemical fertilisers but most commercial fertilisers only contain three active ingredients, typically nitrogen, phosphorus and potassium, not the 50 or so minerals that plants need for optimum health and maximum nutritional value.

Take wheat for example, it is genetically and biologically less nutritious than the wheat my granny used to make a loaf of bread at the weekend. Studies show that modern wheat has 19–28 per cent lower levels of zinc, copper, iron and magnesium than wheat in 1968.

Plus, of course, pesticide residues are often present on crops after harvesting and a cocktail of chemicals are frequently used to clean and preserve fruits and vegetables during processing before being packaged and sent to supermarkets.

This is very different from my granny's day. My granddad had his own veggie patch at the community allotment that supplied us with most of our vegetables. If stocks were running low then granny might buy some carrots at the local greengrocer – they were not washed, uniform and wrapped in plastic. They were loose, covered in dirt and came in all shapes and sizes.

And to top it all off in the 1990s genetically modified (GM) crops entered the food supply chain. While these foods have been approved for human consumption by government agencies, many studies now show the bacterium genetically inserted into crops as an insecticide can colonise the bacteria living in the human digestive tract – killing the good bacteria which modulate serotonin levels in the gut. GM food is ubiquitous in North America and widely used in processed foods and animal feed in the UK (more on that later). I can just imagine what my granny would have said about GM food!

Our Diet Started to Change

Obviously, the changes to food production also started to change our diet. The cost of food started to drop dramatically in the 1980s, and I'll explain why in the next chapter. Technology and innovation also brought us the convenience of the microwave. The traditional range that my granny used to make her delicious pea and ham soup, hearty casseroles and yummy home-made bread and biscuits, as well as keeping the kitchen cosy in winter, was replaced by smaller electric ovens or a short zap in the microwave. Microwave ownership rapidly spread across Britain and the US as did new products to put in them. The first chilled ready meals started to appear in supermarkets. These quick 'heat and eat' processed meals became popular with time-poor women struggling to juggle home and work commitments. But these new food products also contained highly processed ingredients and lacked nutritional value. They also contained new additives and preservatives which were not previously part of our diet. Today we eat, on average, 4kg of these food additives every year.

These new ingredients were included for a variety of reasons but mainly to prolong the shelf life of the product and to make the processed food taste better. The most common flavour enhancer is monosodium glutamate (MSG) and it can be found in all sorts of products including Chinese food, canned vegetables, soups and processed meat. In 1960 we consumed just 12g a year of this artificial flavour enhancer. By 2000 the average person consumed 500g of MSG – that's a 4000 per cent increase in the space of just four decades. MSG may make your beef and black bean sauce tastier but it's an excitotoxin – meaning it causes your brain cells to become overexcited and fire uncontrollably, leading to cell death. MSG is therefore a neurotoxin which kills brain cells in the hypothalamus.

You might be thinking, 'OK, but we've got billions of brain cells so killing off a few with a tasty smoked sausage or convenient bowl of tomato soup every now and again isn't going to make me mad or fat!' On its own, probably not – but cumulatively, together with all the other changes to our diet, and our physical and mental health soon begins to deteriorate. The reason MSG is so dangerous, especially for mental health, is that the hypothalamus plays an important role in linking the nervous system to the endocrine system via the pituitary gland and has a profound impact on regulating metabolism and mood – both essential when we want to avoid being fat or mad!

Oh, and if you think you can check the product labelling for MSG so you can avoid it – good luck! MSG has over 40 other names so that food manufacturers can disguise when it's being added to their products. My granny and millions like her never ate ready meals because they simply didn't exist. And frankly even if they did she wouldn't have been able to afford them. So she didn't have to worry about additives and preservatives and whether she recognised 40 different names for MSG – none of which she would have been able to pronounce!

In my granny's day a chocolate biscuit was for special occasions only. I still remember ferreting around her house looking for the secret stash of Jaffa cakes – usually to be found in the spin dryer! Today we don't need to hunt for our sugar fix or wait for special occasions – we consume 44kg of sugar every year. That's about the weight of an average 12-year-old child – in sugar!

We eat one-third less vegetables and two-thirds less fish (the main source of omega-3) than we did 50 years ago. Organ meat, such as liver and kidneys, are loaded with vitamins and minerals and has the highest concentration of naturally occurring vitamin D of any food group, but organ meats have massively fallen out of fashion. Most British and North American offal is currently exported to mainland Europe and Far Eastern countries as consumers in anglicised nations now prefer steaks, ground beef and chicken breasts.

The staple diet of meat and two vegetables my grandparents routinely enjoyed have been replaced by quick, convenient but often nutritionally devoid pizza, pasta and processed meats. Pickled and fermented vegetables that are high in probiotics have all but disappeared from our dinner tables – ask a kid today what piccalilli is and they'll probably think it is a circus in London! And yet pre and probiotics are essential for brain health as they keep the gut healthy and good bacteria helps produce serotonin in the gut.

When my granny wanted a bacon sandwich she knew where the bacon came from, she baked her own bread and slathered it in lashings of butter. Today we have no idea where the bacon comes from – we hope it wasn't reared in one of those awful metal crates but don't really give it much thought as it crisps up under the grill. Even if we decide to fry our bacon it almost certainly isn't in lard and the butter on our sandwich has been replaced by low-fat spread. Vegetable oils have replaced saturated fats for cooking. You might be wondering, 'But, surely that's good – right?' No, not really because soybean, sunflower, corn and canola oils contain very high amounts of omega-6 fatty acids. Studies show that our body fat stores of linoleic acid (the most common omega-6 fat) have increased by over 300 per cent in the past 50 years. The coconut oil and animal fats used to cook our popcorn at the movies and fish 'n' chips from the local chippie have now been replaced with chemically modified vegetable oils.

Again, you may be tempted to think this isn't a problem and are wondering why I'm getting my 'knickers in a twist' as we say in Scotland. The reason is simple. These new 'healthier' oils and spreads were not designed because the companies wanted to make us healthier – they were created because these massive food giants had huge quantities of waste by-product from their primary business that they needed to deal with. They could either get rid of it, which is time consuming and costly, or they could convert it into another product and sell that to us too. Back those products with millions in advertising to convince us they are healthy and voilà – billions more in revenue.

Take corn as an example; in the US alone they grow something in the region of 333 million tonnes of corn a year. Not only is there an oversupply of corn but its production creates a massive amount of waste product – the stalk of the corn. Thirty-three million tonnes of corn creates A LOT of useless corn stalks to get rid of. In traditional farming, certainly for barley production, the waste stalks are bailed up as straw and used as bedding for the animals in winter. But for massive agri-food businesses that's time consuming and there is no money in it. So they have found multiple ways to make additional products, not only from the corn itself but from the waste by-product too. High fructose corn syrup (HFCS) is an artificial sweetener made from a highly secret process using the corn stalk. HFCS is used in all sorts of products including soft drinks and yet it has been linked to a wide range of diseases and disorders.

Research is now proving that my granny's use of fats and oils was the healthy approach. Everyone knows what's in butter – milk, a little salt and very little else. Do you know how some of those vegetable, corn or soy oils are made? No – only the scientists in secret laboratories know that. And yet often these products are marketed as 'natural' or 'healthy'. Can we really call a product that is literally resurrected from a waste by-product with zero nutritional value and turned into something else through chemical alchemy natural? No.

We were first warned about our fat intake in the 1970s and again in the 1980s and yet an Anglo-American study concluded that no such advice would have been made based on modern-day clinical trials (which are themselves flawed as I'll soon explain). The study published in online journal *Open Heart* concluded, 'It seems incomprehensible that dietary advice was introduced to 220 million Americans and 56 million UK citizens, given the contrary results from a small number of unhealthy men.' No wonder none of us are losing weight on a low-fat diet!

A Harvard study published in *Lancet Diabetes & Endocrinology* compiling information from 53 previous trials compared the effectiveness of low-fat diets and research data from more than 68,000 adults and concluded that what we have been told as 'fact' for nearly 40-plus years is just not true.

Obviously, I'm not advocating you start adding butter to everything and going ballistic on the chips but between false data and corporations hijacking the narrative so we will buy their 'Frankenfood' it's not really very surprising that so many of us are mad or fat!

Our Medication Started to Change

In addition to the food production and dietary changes, a new generation of antidepressants hit the market in the 1980s and 1990s, including selective serotonin reuptake inhibitors (SSRIs). SSRIs such as Prozac (fluoxetine), Paxil and Seroxat (paroxetine) and Zoloft (sertraline) all contain high amounts of either fluoride or chlorine, both of which, along with bromine, are what I call 'bad halogens' (more on them in chapter 5). Bad halogens are neurotoxins and endocrine disruptors which displace iodine in the body leading to thyroid dysfunction. Plus these bad halogens are now ubiquitous in our life – they can be in our drinking water, our food, the furniture in our homes, the personal care products we use as well as medicine such as antidepressants.

Let me ask you – what do you consider an acceptable number of side effects for a drug? Ten? Fifty maybe – so long as it works. What about 2,000? How would you feel about medicine if it had 2,000 side effects? The number of listed side effects associated with taking antidepressants is staggering:

- Prozac – 1,817 side effects
- Zoloft – 2,194 side effects
- Paxil – 2,497 side effects

Weight gain is also a common side effect for SSRIs – causing food cravings, especially for carbohydrates and sugars. SSRIs also impact metabolism. Unsurprisingly, the rise in antidepressant prescriptions is mirrored by the rise in obesity rates. Between 1990 and 2010 there has been a 400 per cent increase in people taking happy pills and antidepressant use and obesity has been intrinsically linked ever since. Of course, the two are inextricably linked. Sure, some people genuinely don't mind being a bit overweight but I've yet to meet anyone who enjoyed being depressed. If on top of being depressed you pile on weight that's absolutely not going to help you feel better about yourself!

Today antidepressants are the most common prescription drug in the US. And almost 800,000 Scots take antidepressants – over 518,000 are women. The highest antidepressant usage in Scotland is in the Greater Glasgow and Clyde area – where diet is notoriously poor. Historically this is also where the sugar came off the boats from the Caribbean and it is still where almost all the Scottish sugar refineries are located today. These two factors are not a coincidence and we'll discuss the negative effect sugar has on the brain in chapter 6.

What makes all this even worse is that the explosion of

antidepressant use is based on erroneous data. For example, Prozac worked for some people but only when it was administered with a tranquilliser so that they did not attempt suicide. However that piece of information, which you could argue was pretty crucial, was omitted from the clinical trial data. You don't have to be Einstein to realise that it could have been the tranquilliser not the drug that was having the positive effect but that was simply ignored and Prozac is now one of the most prescribed drugs on the planet – making billions for the manufacturer.

Plus SSRI drugs were developed on the premise that depression is caused by a serotonin imbalance in the brain but there is no medical test to prove this. Antidepressants do nothing to solve the root problem of mental illness and a growing body of evidence now shows that depression is a biological disorder caused by micronutrient deficiencies in the diet. While serotonin is a key neurotransmitter in the brain, 90 per cent of serotonin is synthesised in the gut and therefore very susceptible to what we eat (because it ends up in the gut).

The Perfect Mad Fat Storm

All these various changes have created a 'perfect storm' and the mad fat epidemic is the result.

Some 60 per cent of Western women go on a diet every year. For many this is a soul-destroying few months that doesn't even work. And it doesn't work because often the dieter is eating low-fat or low-calorie ready meals – a market worth £2 billion in the UK alone. Time-pressed women who don't have time for breakfast are reaching instead for the 'healthy' low-fat cereal breakfast bar – many of which are endorsed by popular slimming or cereal brands. It doesn't matter that a skinny girl in a red dress is advertising it – eating a chocolate-coated granola bar loaded with sugar is NOT going to help you lose weight or feel energised.

Just think about this for a moment…in 2014, the global market for weight loss products was valued at over $586 billion.

If those products worked then we would all be happily skipping around in little red dresses and yet we are not. Why? Because those companies don't really want us to get slim and healthy otherwise it's goodbye $586 billion – what they want is to sell us hope so we will continue to buy them and keep their massive profits rolling in. So ask yourself, do these companies really want to help us lose weight and feel better or are they simply happy to sell us the illusion?

The low-fat, low-salt, low-cholesterol diets promoted by Western governments mean that more and more women are buying foods high in carbohydrates and new 'healthy eating' products. But, when manufacturers remove fat from processed foods it is substituted with chemically modified additives – refined sugars, starches (which turn to sugar in the body) and other synthetic ingredients which mimic the effects of fat during manufacture. Also, more and more artificial flavour enhancers and preservatives with unpronounceable names are added to counteract the lack of salt – which authorities are now telling us is bad for us too.

Clever supermarket food marketing often encourages us to buy the wrong foods packaged as the right foods and this is contributing to the mad fat epidemic. These foods are making us fat and foggy while pretending to make us thin and energetic. Even if you buy fresh fruit and vegetables and are genuinely eating the 'right food' the mass production of many of our key food groups has led to a radical reduction in micronutrients. Today we simply don't consume enough vitamins and minerals for optimum brain health.

Take magnesium, for example, it is essential for mental health and good sleep and yet statistics now show that 80 per cent of people eating a Western diet are chronically deficient in magnesium. Depending on the demographic group studied, anywhere between 40 and 60 per cent of the population are deficient in vitamin D. Between 1971 and 2001 iodine consumption in the US dropped by 50 per cent. Most schoolgirls and pregnant women in the UK are iodine deficient and yet even a mild deficiency in iodine impairs mental function. Thirty per cent of us do not consume enough vitamin C. Forty-four per cent of us are deficient in vitamin A. Our bodies may be fat but our brains are starved of vital nutrients! And it is a lack of these micronutrients that is the real root cause of depression and ill health.

Instead of nutrient-rich food we are eating way too much sugar and food additives that are harming our brain. Genetic modification of food and junk food is killing off the good bacteria in our gut which helps to modulate serotonin levels. We are also eating too much omega-6 and not enough omega-3. Add the bad halogens and we have created a 'perfect storm' of contributing factors that are having a devastating impact on our physical and mental health.

I often wonder what my granny and her friends in the tenement buildings of Possilpark would have made of the pickle we've created for ourselves. They were poor and yet ironically their lack of money was instrumental in keeping them incredibly healthy. My granny and her friends didn't have the plethora of choice and convenience foods we have today. And before you panic, I'm not advocating a move back to the 'good old days'. You don't need to be rich, you don't need a private chef or have your meals delivered to your door, and you don't need to visit the gym seven days a week. What you need to do is get educated about the food you're eating and open your eyes to what's really going on.

Part Two
History of the Problem

'We may find in the long run that tinned food is a deadlier weapon than the machine-gun.'

– George Orwell

Chapter 2: The War on Food

'About eighty percent of the food on shelves of supermarkets today didn't exist 100 years ago.'

– Larry McCleary

So how did we create the mad fat epidemic that is now sweeping across North America, the UK, Europe and beyond? Surely, this wasn't some conspiracy or powerful figures plotting the doom of civilisation. Sometimes I really wonder, but no, it's probably not that exciting. Many of the changes were instigated for the right or at least understandable reasons. And, like most things in life, many of the changes boil down to cold hard cash.

In reality, the alterations to food production were a direct result of the Second World War. At the time Britain imported more than 22 million tonnes of food from overseas and was heavily reliant on the boats bringing vital supplies to the UK, usually across the Atlantic.

Part of Rudyard Kipling's poem 'Big Steamers' sets the scene perfectly:

'Oh, where are you going to, all you Big Steamers,
With England's own coal, up and down the salt seas?'
'We are going to fetch you your bread and your butter,
Your beef, pork, and mutton, eggs, apples, and cheese.'
'And where will you fetch it from, all you Big Steamers,
And where shall I write you when you are away?'
'We fetch it from Melbourne, Quebec, and Vancouver,
Address us at Hobart, Hong Kong, and Bombay.'
'But if anything happened to all you Big Steamers,
And suppose you were wrecked up and down the salt sea?'
'Then you'd have no coffee or bacon for breakfast,

And you'd have no muffins or toast for your tea.'

During the Second World War many of these 'Big Steamers' and merchant boats were sunk by the German U-boat fleet. The loss of merchant shipping vessels carrying food and military supplies was often a far greater threat to Britain's survival than German troops invading the UK. After all, if there wasn't enough food people would starve – hardly a comforting thought in the middle of war.

Food rationing was imposed to preserve what little was left or getting through and the Women's Land Army was enlisted to grow as much as possible. Once the war was over the grimness of food rationing was not forgotten. In 1947, the British government passed the Agriculture Act with the express purpose of lowering the amount of food imported into Britain and to promote maximum agricultural productivity. At least if war did ever break out again, British citizens would never be vulnerable to siege or food shortage again.

Introduction of Food Subsidies

Food subsidies were introduced to encourage landowners to put as much of their land as possible into food production. This well-intentioned strategy made sense. The UK needed to be more self-sufficient for the future and the best way to ensure that outcome was to incentivise landowners to produce more food. The problem with financial incentives, as we have witnessed more recently in the green energy sector, is that it distorts effort and some people seek to 'game' the system. Just like subsidies for erecting wind turbines attracted large business into the green energy sector, some landowners sought to capitalise on the lucrative subsidies on offer by ramping up food production. Smaller, traditionally run family farms were bought up by large corporations and large-scale industrial farming began in the UK.

The difference in approach was often stark. Smaller, traditionally run farms are often mixed farms, meaning that the farmer rears a variety of animals and grows a variety of crops to feed those animals through the winter months. Any excess grain, hay, silage or straw for bedding is simply sold to other local farmers. The animals are raised on grass pastures and some, including cattle, are usually wintered indoors. Cattle don't like being wet or cold! The manure collected from the animals during the winter months is then spread on the fields as fertiliser helping to return organic matter to the land as well as the 50 or so minerals needed for healthy soil. Crops are rotated, in other words one field would grow barley one year and potatoes or grass the next. The following year the same field may be used to grow turnips or kale. Growing different crops in successive years reduces soil erosion and increases soil fertility. Because each crop requires a different combination of nutrients to grow, growing different crops also allows the soil to rejuvenate between growing cycles and this is further assisted by the manure from the animals as organic fertiliser. Crop rotation also reduces pathogens and pests that may like one crop but not another. Traditionally the emphasis is on quality not quantity, fields tended to be quite small and hedgerows were intact, further aiding wildlife diversification.

Subsidies changed all that for vast swathes of the countryside. Large landowners and food production companies removed the hedgerows to make larger fields so that it was easier and quicker to harvest using the new machinery. Although crop rotation can increase yield it also increases workload. However, chemical fertilisers could ensure higher yield without the higher workload.

In terms of food production – subsidies worked. In 1938–9 the output of British agriculture was valued at £2.5 million, £1.4 million of which was exported. In 1951 output was over £100 million, half of which was exported. Food production in the UK had increased dramatically – Britain was safe. The problem, of course, is that taxpayer-funded subsidies were creating a huge incentive to produce more and more foods, so it wasn't long before Britain was producing too much food, leading to 'milk lakes' and 'grain or butter mountains' – vast amounts of food rotting in huge chilled containers, barns or unused aircraft hangars. But this was largely considered an acceptable consequence of preserving food security.

The same thing also happened in the US where government funding drove overproduction of corn, wheat and soy, ignoring all the other cereals and grains previously produced by farmers. One hundred years ago British and American farmers cultivated over 50 types of cereals and grains; today that has reduced to three main ones. In the US the three are corn, soy and wheat and in the UK they are wheat, rapeseed and barley.

But these changes didn't just impact milk, butter, grains and cereals, they also had a big impact on meat production. The government also wanted to reduce our reliance on imported meat so farmers were encouraged to utilise new technology. 'New technology' included new animal feedstuffs designed to fatten the animal quicker. It was a new feedstuff that, unbeknown to the farmers that used it, contained other animal by-products, that caused the UK BSE or mad cow crisis in the 1990s. Why anyone thought it was a good idea to feed herbivores meat and bonemeal from another animal is beyond me. Like so much of the food we eat today, this raw ingredient was, of course, disguised and added to other ingredients so it looked like regular cattle feed. The other 'new technology' that made a big difference was new vaccines and antibiotics. When Scottish scientist Alexander Fleming discovered penicillin it didn't just revolutionise human health, it had a huge impact on animal health too. These two technologies in combination helped to fuel intensive livestock production.

New foodstuff and increased antibiotic use

Remember the 'good guys' and the 'bad guys' I referred to earlier – the 'good guys' raise their animals outside in summer where they can enjoy lush grass, plenty of open space and sunshine. In winter cattle are brought back into sheds and barns. They still have plenty of room to move around, can go outside if they want but can also bed down at night on clean straw out of the winter elements. For the 'good guys' animal welfare is paramount, not because their government tells them it is but because they are genuine farmers and animal caretakers. To people who have lived or grown up in a city their whole life and don't necessarily appreciate the 24/7 commitment required to be a traditional farmer, the idea of raising an animal to kill it for meat can seem completely bonkers, but to the 'good guys' it's the natural cycle of life. They care about their animals and they bend over backwards to ensure the life an animal has is a healthy and happy one. This is why we need to champion the 'good guys' and support them in our own communities.

The 'bad guys' focus instead on factory farming where large numbers of animals are squashed up together in dark barns, they never see the sky and are often caged. For example, pigs were often raised in 'pig crates' that restricted their movement. Thankfully, these crates were banned in the UK in 1999 and in 2013 in Europe but they are still used elsewhere. Normally these cramped and poor conditions would cause disease which is why new vaccines made factory farming possible.

Although this type of intensive farming for pigs and cattle is on the decrease it still happens in mainland Europe, as farmers resist implementing costly changes, and it is still happening in the US. Plus, unfortunately much of the damage has already been done to our food supply. Wider use of vaccines and antibiotics plus extensive use of pesticides and herbicides has already changed the chemistry and nutritional value of our food. If chemicals are in the animal or plant then they will be on our plate and end up inside us. And, elevated chemical, hormones, heavy metal and antibiotic residue in the food we eat is damaging our mental and physical well-being.

Now, you might be thinking, 'What's she banging on about? What does it matter if we consume a tiny amount of antibiotic residues in our food, or breathe in the odd particle or two?' Trust me, it matters. And it matters a great deal if you are currently mad, fat or both!

Although Fleming's discovery of penicillin in 1928 paved the way for antibiotics, penicillin wasn't purified and mass-produced until 1944. A year later, while giving his Nobel Prize acceptance speech, Fleming gave a stark warning about the overuse of antibiotics saying:

I would like to sound one note of warning. Although penicillin is to all intents and purposes non-poisonous so there is no need to worry about giving an overdose and poisoning the patient, it is not difficult to make microbes resistant to penicillin in the laboratory by exposing them to concentrations not sufficient to kill them, and the same thing has occasionally happened in the body. The time may come when penicillin can be bought by anyone in the shops. Then there is the danger that the ignorant man may easily underdose himself and by exposing his microbes to the non-lethal quantities of the drug make them resistant.

We clearly listened to the 'non-poisonous', 'no fear of overdosing' part of Fleming's speech but we universally ignored the 'overuse leads to resistance' part. Antibiotics were astonishingly successful for human and animal health but they have been *seriously* overused.

Until quite recently intensively reared chicken and pigs had access to water that contained antibiotics – as a precautionary measure against infection. In the US, factory-farmed pigs, cows and chickens are all still reared intensively with a heavy reliance on antibiotics which then ends up in our food.

Ten million kilograms of antibiotics are used in animal agriculture each year in the US alone. A study published in 2015 by Texas Tech University showed that DNA from antibiotic-resistant bacteria is spreading from cattle feedlots across the US through the air. The Texan scientists looked at more than three-quarters of all cattle on US feedlots – a total of 8.24 million cattle. The scientists extracted DNA from the particle matter bound to the air filters located both upwind and downwind of the feedlots and they detected the presence of nine antibiotic-resistant genes in the filters. Not only was the cattle, and therefore the meat, antibiotic resistant but most of these feedlots were located in the southern High Plains, known for dust storms. So this particle matter was being spread in the wind to further pollute land and water systems. This report suggested that the so-called superbugs threatening humans can be traced back to the overuse of antibiotics in animals.

Falling Prices and Failing Health

Of course, when supply of anything goes up the price usually comes down. This was good news for ordinary people as their weekly food shopping bill started to fall. This certainly helped people like my grandparents who were used to spending a large part of their income on food. Unfortunately, the focus on quantity over quality had a knock-on effect on our health. And for the most part we still don't actually realise it!

Although the consumer appeared to benefit from the reduction in food cost we still paid a price – usually in our health. The big winners were the large landowners – the men who sat in the House of Lords, presiding over government policy, while raking in hundreds of thousands of pounds, sometimes millions from the new Acts that they helped pass.

In the UK most of Britain's agricultural subsidies fall into the hands of corporations, despite the fact that there are over 221,000 registered farming operations. The prices that small farmers currently get for their produce is also so low that subsidies now form a substantial part of the income of the 'good guys'. Cheap farm gate prices create a form of corporate welfare with public funds in the form of farm subsidies going straight into the pocket of traders, processors and retailers. The only farming operations reaping the benefit are the major farming operations – like the barley barons in East Anglia, the megadairies and the absentee landlords cashing in from their vast estates. Subsidies are based on volume of production – so the big producers get the most. What so many of us don't realise is that the people producing our food are usually paid a pittance for it. This is especially true if it is bought by large supermarket chains with a lot of buying muscle. We may see a beef joint on the supermarket shelves and think, 'Wow that's a bit pricey', but the farmer wasn't paid that price; they were paid a fraction of that price and the retailer takes the lion's share.

It is the food processors and retailers that are the big winners – because of subsidies they are able to buy food from the producers at rock-bottom prices and add a considerable margin before selling it on to us. It is the middlemen that are benefiting from farm subsidies not the farmers themselves – at least not unless the farmer owns thousands of acres. Today, through the acquisition of small family-run dairies, three multinational companies dominate British milk production and you can count on one hand the number of corporations who control meat processing. These food processing giants have contracts with the main UK supermarkets – and between them they control what we eat, how it is produced and how much it costs.

In the US too, subsidies have led to the same consolidation of the agricultural industry by huge agri-food businesses. A handful of multinational corporations now control the American food supply. Just four companies control meat production in the US. Ninety per cent of US soybean crop and 80 per cent of the corn and cotton grown in the US use Monsanto's genetically modified seeds. We will talk about GM food later.

Supermarket growth on both sides of the Atlantic has seen the near extinction of local greengrocers. There is nowhere, except perhaps farmers' markets, where we can buy dirty vegetables – now they are washed, sprayed with various chemicals and packed in plastic. My granddad bought his meat direct from the farmer but now even traditional butchers are struggling to compete with the supermarkets. And bakers and fishmongers are also struggling to keep their heads above water. Back in the 1970s Tesco was struggling and Walmart was a regional grocer with just 125 stores. In 2016, these grocers dominate the food industry in the UK and US, alongside the agri-food giants. It is them and their direct competitors who carve up the market, control our food and influence our governments.

Their goal is profit and our food and our health has suffered as a result.

Big Food is Almost Always Bad Food

Today a handful of faceless corporations have grown into global giants and have successfully hijacked our food supply for profit. Boards of directors serving shareholders now dominate the decision-making and this quest to constantly increase profit has changed the way we produce and process food. These global giants exert a huge amount of influence on our governments and policymakers through the lobby. Lobbying is basically legalised bribery where business or other vested interests pay lobbyists to get to the ear of policymakers and influence decisions that could potentially impact their business – either positively or negatively.

Take the major health issue of cholesterol as an example. In my granny's day no one was talking about cholesterol. Today *everyone* is talking about cholesterol. We are told that we need to monitor our cholesterol levels. We're even encouraged to eat certain low-fat spreads to help. What we are not told is why. The reason is money, plain and simple.

There are two types of cholesterol – good cholesterol (HDL) and bad cholesterol (LDL). And statins are a family of medication that are used to regulate bad cholesterol in the blood. In 2004 the US-based National Cholesterol Education Program (NCEP) recommended that previously acceptable levels of cholesterol be lowered. The NCEP is an expert panel assembled by the National Institute of Health so what they say must be right. Right? Apparently not. A scientific assessment of the NCEP's recommendations published in 2006 revealed, 'No high quality clinical evidence to support current treatment goals for [LDL] cholesterol.' That study also stated that the recommended practice of adjusting statin dosages to achieve the new recommended cholesterol levels was not scientifically proven to be beneficial or safe.

Hang on, if there was no benefit from these drugs, they were unsafe and there was no evidence that our cholesterol levels were too high in the first place, why was the recommendation made?

Could it have been the fact that eight out of the nine members of the NCEP's 'expert' panel had financial links to companies that manufactured statin drugs? Just think about that for a moment…What better way to sell more drugs and make more money than by inventing a problem that didn't actually exist. By lowering the acceptable levels of bad cholesterol the industry immediately created a new market of consumers for their statin drugs. Of course, by the time this clear conflict of interest was discovered and made public, the lower levels had passed into medical 'fact' and now we are bombarded with cholesterol-lowering drugs and food products to combat a problem that often doesn't even exist.

In early 2016 NHS cardiologist Dr Aseem Malhotra joined forces with six eminent doctors, including Sir Richard Thompson, the Queen's personal doctor for 21 years, in call-ing for an urgent public inquiry into drug companies' murky practices. Dr Malhotra claims the full trial data on statins hasnever been published. He is particularly critical of the dramaticrecent increase of the prescription of statins to millions of people – drawing attention to the lack of evidence of their efficacy and the same questionable conflict of interest detailed above.

To be clear, I'm not saying that high levels of bad cholesterol is a good thing – it's not – but maybe what is considered high isn't really that high at all and a few changes to diet and lifestyle would do significantly more to benefit your health than taking potentially dangerous statins.

Unfortunately, this type of scenario is rife. In the UK 138 officials responsible for advising or making decisions on drugs adopted by the NHS are receiving payments from pharmaceutical firms. 'Big pharma' paid doctors and officials across the NHS £30 million in 2015 and spent another £10 million sponsoring their attendance at events. When you consider that the NHS spends over £15 billion per year on prescription drugs – an amount which is increasing 8 per cent year on year – it's easy to see why spending a mere £40 million in the hope of influencing lucrative decisions is a smart business decision by pharmaceutical companies. That's a pretty awesome return on investment.

More than one in three members of the Department of Health panel which oversees NHS medicine procurement receives money from 'big pharma'. Drug companies pay these government officials £1,000 for every NHS panel meeting they attend on top of other 'consulting fees' for their work on behalf of the drug companies.

The point is that people in power, Potentially driven by self-interest, are making decisions on our behalf and we don't even know about it. Whether through incentivising an expert panel to make business-friendly recommendations or through lobbying politicians, it is very clear that decisions are being made that benefit the few over the many. In the UK former Prime Minister David Cameron promised to 'sort it out'. In his 'Rebuilding Trust in Politics' speech delivered in February 2010 he said, 'We all know how it works. The lunches, the hospitality, the quiet word in the ear, the ex-ministers and ex-advisers for hire, helping big business find the right way to get its way. We don't know who is meeting whom. We don't know whether any favours are being exchanged. We don't know which outside interests are wielding unhealthy influence. This isn't a minor issue with minor consequences. Commercial interests – not to mention government contracts worth hundreds of billions of pounds – are potentially at stake. I believe that secret corporate lobbying...goes to the heart of why people are so fed up with politics. It arouses people's worst fears and suspicions about how our political system works, with money buying power, power fishing for money and a cosy club at the top making decisions in their own interest. It is increasingly clear that lobbying in this country is getting out of control. We can't go on like this.'

But we are still going on like this. In the US over the last five years alone the 200 most politically active companies spent $5.8 billion influencing the US government and those same companies got $4.4 trillion in taxpayer support. That's a massive return on investment, and it's only the top 200 most politically active companies. That said, at least in the US the lobbying is upfront and relatively open. In the UK it's all usually done behind closed doors and nobody gets to know about it.

Buying muscle and food adulteration

Because of their buying power big business dictates price and product specifications to farmers. In 2015 celebrity chef Hugh Fearnley-Whittingstall kicked off his 'War on Waste' in a TV documentary. In the programme he spoke to a family of parsnip farmers who had asked Morrisons – one of the main supermarkets in the UK – to increase the maximum permissible size for parsnips from 70mm at the base (2.8in) to 75mm (3in), but the supermarket refused. To be clear, there is absolutely nothing wrong with the parsnips and yet the supplier was forced to dump 20 tonnes per week just because they were slightly larger than the arbitrary specifications laid down by the powerful supermarket. When people are still dying of starvation in many parts of the world and over a million people are using food banks in the UK, the fact that we are dumping hundreds of thousands of tonnes of edible fruit and vegetables alone is an absolute disgrace. Plus the argument behind GM food is that we need to pursue GM food options if we stand any chance of feeding the escalating number of people on the planet. Maybe if we didn't waste so much perfectly good food because it doesn't meet some stupid rule we could feed everyone just fine!

Supermarket giants have huge legal teams fighting their battles and their buyers are trained to beat suppliers into submission on price. In the US the roles are somewhat reversed because, apart from Wal-mart, the food processors control the retailers to a certain extent. But the outcome is the same – someone in the middle is making all the money and those at either end ('good guy' farmers and consumers) are suffering.

Food processors are squeezed for greater margin and they in turn will often then squeeze the grower or farmer. And when those food manufacturers can't be squeezed any more they are often forced into desperate measures, such as mislabelling products or food adulteration.

If you were in the UK in 2013 you will probably remember the 'horsemeat scandal' when certain Tesco 'beefburgers' were found to contain 29 per cent horsemeat instead of beef. Other food manufacturers and retailers were also involved. Social media went crazy with horsemeat jokes but it was no laughing matter. This is the sort of food adulteration that happens when suppliers and producers are constantly squeezed to make more money or reduce costs. Philip Clarke, Tesco CEO at the time, made a public apology and the retailer promised to put in place a 'world-class traceability system' to ensure this would never happen again. Months later Tesco were caught again – this time selling Dutch pork and passing it off as British – and in 2014 they admitted their pork sausages contained chicken. As of 2016, Tesco are yet to introduce a traceability system and although there has been several executive staff changes at the retailer and it is under investigation for accounting irregularities, it is business as usual on their sourcing policies. They are, for example, still buying some of their beef from the beef processing giant that supplied the horse burgers. Interestingly, the Tesco beef supplier who supplied those burgers was also the main beef supplier to Sainsbury's – another leading British supermarket. But no horsemeat was found in Sainsbury's beefburgers, indicating they were probably not driven so hard on price and could therefore afford to deliver what was asked for without compromising on quality.

What makes matters worse is that DEFRA (Department for Environment, Food and Rural Affairs) at Westminster were made fully aware of the mass discrepancies in the British beef supply chain in 2012 – long before the story hit the headlines. They considered it a 'matter for industry' and were no doubt encouraged to maintain that position by lobbyists working for deep-pocketed companies who did not want or welcome government intervention in their food supply chain. Plus, of course, Tesco employs over 300,000 people in the UK, so maybe that had a bearing on their decision to sweep the horsemeat information under the carpet. Luckily, the Irish government blew the whistle in January 2013 – despite the potential risk to their own beef sector which is a key contributor to their GDP. By early 2016 none of the big food companies involved in 'horsegate' had been prosecuted.

This type of activity is known as food fraud. Food producers add cheaper horsemeat to their '100% beefburgers', cheaper syrup to honey or even add food colouring to turn cheap sunflower oil into extra virgin olive oil. Food is often deliberately mislabelled with cheaper species of fish being sold as haddock or cod, fish is often also advertised as 'line caught' when it's caught by trawlers or advertised as 'wild' when it's actually farmed. But food adulteration is not a new phenomenon. In the nineteenth century plaster of Paris was used as a sugar substitute. Yes – the stuff used to make a plaster cast, or as we say in Scotland a 'stookie', when you break a leg. Chalk was added to flour, sawdust was added to dough, alum was added to loaves to make them whiter and strychnine was added to improve the taste of watered-down beer. By the beginning of the nineteenth century the use of these foreign, often toxic, substances in manufactured foods became so common that shoppers began to develop a taste for the adulterated products – preferring this 'fake food' to the real thing. Demand for these often dangerous products soared. Fast forward 200 years and nothing much has changed other than the fact that food adulteration is now often legal! Producers may not be adding alum, plaster of Paris and strychnine to our food – but they are adding bread improvers, artificial flavours such as MSG, colourants, fillers and preservatives to boost profits. And just like our ancestors hundreds of years ago, we've grown to like the taste of E-numbers, acidifying agents, stabilisers, emulsifiers, raising agents, artificial sweeteners, azo dyes and industrially hydrogenated fats. So much so that many of us are now hooked on them and regularly consume products masquerading as food with little or no nutritional value. Some are even toxic!

The Cumulative Negative Impact of the War on Food

Change is a normal and positive part of life. We have made huge strides in so many areas and food is definitely one of those areas. The 1947 Agriculture Act did fulfil its brief and provided food security, but the knock-on effect of incentivising and commercialising food production has created untold damage elsewhere.

Individually many of these little shifts may not seem that big a deal but collectively they are having a profound impact on our physical and mental well-being. Our diet is almost unrecognisable to the diet our grandparents ate.

Part of the reason that we have been slow to connect the dots between this change in diet and our well-being is that the changes themselves have been slow. When something catastrophic and sudden happens, it's easy to track back and find the cause, but when we have experienced a slow and steady decline in our health with increasing allergies, a plethora of stomach disorders, rising obesity and mental health problems, it's not as easy or obvious to point the finger at one cause. The truth is there is not one cause because the changes to our diet have been several – not just in the way food is produced, but by how it's processed and packaged too.

Taken collectively this war on our food has radically altered what we eat and has inadvertently created the mad fat epidemic.

Chapter 3: A Brief History of Medicine

'Whenever a doctor cannot do good, he must be kept from doing harm.'

– Hippocrates

Adding fuel to the mad fat fire are the changes in medicine – specifically the changes to mental health medicine.

In 1431, during one of the most famous trials in history, Joan of Arc testified to hearing voices in her head. Apparently they told her to deliver France from the invading English and establish Charles VII as the rightful heir to the French throne. Almost 600 years later doctors have 'diagnosed' Joan with a wide range of mental disorders ranging from schizophrenia, to bipolar disorder, to epilepsy. Today, it's likely that Joan would be prescribed psychotropic drugs to deal with her 'disorder'. What a loss to France and history that would have been!

There is little doubt that the tremendous breakthroughs in our understanding of health and the treatment of disease have saved millions of lives and improved the quality of life for many millions more. But, often these innovations have also had significant unintended consequences.

We Stopped Taking Responsibility

For a start, these medical breakthroughs and innovations allowed us to outsource responsibility for our own health.

In my grandparents' day, you needed to pay to see the doctor; most people were fairly poor so they engaged in preventative medicine – before there was even a term for it! With the advent of wonder drugs, like antibiotics that could cure a vast range of diseases, people became less concerned with prevention because if worst came to worst at least there was a magic pill that would make them better. This mindset has gathered pace ever since and we have become major pill poppers. In the US, pharmaceutical companies will offer free trials of their medication via TV adverts without really going into detail about what the pill actually does and yet people clearly phone up for their free sample!

It's easy to see the attraction of popping a pill to solve our problems but that approach definitely has side effects. Our overuse of antibiotics in animals and humans is a classic example. Antibiotics revolutionised human health – they have saved millions of lives and their benefit to humanity can't be underestimated.

But, we have used them far too often for conditions or ailments that really didn't require their use. Every sniffle, cough and splutter was treated with a prescription of antibiotics. Of course, they were so effective that the patient soon began to feel better and stopped taking the medication, thereby allowing the infection to mutate in the body and become antibiotic resistant. Even though it clearly states that we need to finish the full course of antibiotics when we are prescribed them, most of us don't. This coupled with the overuse of antibiotics in animal rearing has resulted in superbugs such as MRSA that do not respond to antibiotics at all. In 2015, Mark Baker, director of clinical practice at the National Institute for Health and Care Excellence (NICE), warned that doctors write 10 million needless antibiotic prescriptions each year. This overuse means that antibiotics may soon be obsolete – an outcome that will have Fleming spinning in his grave. What a waste of a phenomenal drug. Of course, antibiotics are still essential for critical care and operations but their impact has been reduced by overuse. We urgently need to move away from antibiotics for anything except emergency care.

There is now way too much antibiotic residue in our bodies. On top of the antibiotics we may have taken as a prescription from our doctor, that residue is now being constantly 'topped up' because of the food we eat. Interestingly, the link between antibiotic overuse and mental health is beginning to emerge.

Conservatively there are about 1,000 different varieties of microbes coexisting harmoniously within a typical healthy person's gut. In fact, the average adult carries up to five pounds of bacteria. Ninety per cent of serotonin, so crucial for mood and mental well-being, is created in the gut from healthy gut bacteria. Healthy good bacteria, known as probiotics, also regulate dopamine levels and 'talk to the brain' through the immune system or parts of the nervous system. The problem is that antibiotics don't discriminate between good bacteria and bad. They don't just kill the bad bacteria – they kill *all* the gut bacteria. According to Dr Martin Blaser, Chairman of the Department of Medicine at New York University's Langone Medical Center, overuse of antibiotics may be changing our entire bacterial make-up. In a paper published in *Nature*, one of the most prestigious medical journals in the US, Blaser cited evidence that antibiotics may permanently change the beneficial bacteria in our gut.

A study co-led by researchers at the Universitat de València reveals that antibiotics produce changes in the microbial and metabolic patterns of the gut. For the first time this research showed that gut bacteria presents a lower capacity to produce proteins, as well as deficiencies in key activities, during and after the antibiotic treatment. Specifically, the study suggests that the gut microbiota show less capacity to absorb iron, digest certain foods and produce essential molecules. Iron is essential for mental (and physical) well-being because iron carries oxygen throughout our bloodstream. Low levels of iron can reduce the oxygen in the blood which can cause the development of psychological problems such as anxiety, panic attacks and extreme mental fatigue. If we are iron deficient we are also unable to digest certain foods, which also affects how much micronutrients we absorb – the vitamins and minerals essential for keeping us healthy.

In a separate study in 2013, low levels of healthy gut bacteria were linked to mental health issues such as anxiety, schizophrenia and autism. The study published in *Nutritional Neuroscience* from the Great Plains Laboratory showed that HPHPA levels – a chemical by-product of clostridia bacteria (bad bacteria) – are much higher in autistic children. The study showed that after treating teenagers who suffer from obsessive-compulsive disorder (OCD) and attention deficit hyperactivity disorder (ADHD) for six months with high-strength probiotics their symptoms began to disappear and after a year they were completely gone! Just stop and think about that for a moment…These conditions affect millions of people worldwide, causing stress and anxiety to them and the people who love them. Drug companies get richer from endless prescriptions and yet increasing our probiotics, either through improved diet and/or supplements, is much more effective and could cure these conditions.

And finally, McMaster University in Canada published the results of their research project in the *Journal of Communicative and Integrative Biology* in 2010 showing a link between gut bacteria and mental health. Scientists compared the behaviour of normal eight-week-old mice to mice of the same age that had been stripped of their natural gut bacteria. The mice without any gut bacteria showed higher levels of the stress hormone cortisol and were exhibiting risk-taking behaviour. Granted, I'm not exactly sure what risk-taking behaviour in a mouse looks like, but in all seriousness the lack of bacteria was shown to alter levels of a brain chemical called BDNF which is linked to depression and anxiety in humans.

Commercialisation of Medicine

The second big change was the commercialisation of medicine. New innovations created new opportunities to make money and, boy, did the big pharmaceutical companies coin it in!

In her book *The Truth About Drug Companies*, author Marcia Angell MD, who is also incidentally the first woman to serve as editor-in-chief of the prestigious *New England Journal of*

Medicine, reported that in 2002 the profits earned by the top ten drug companies in the Fortune 500 (the richest companies in the US) were greater than the profit of the other 490 Fortune 500 companies combined!

Figure 3.1: World's largest pharmaceutical firms

World's Largest Pharmaceutical Firms				
Company	Total Revenue ($bn)	R&D Spend ($bn)	Sales & Marketing Spend ($bn)	Profit ($bn)
Johnson & Johnson (US)	71.3	8.2	17.5	13.8
Novartis (Swiss)	58.8	9.9	14.6	9.2
Pfizer (US)	51.6	6.6	11.4	22.0
Hoffman-La Roche (Swiss)	50.3	9.3	9.0	12.0
Sanofi (France)	44.4	6.3	9.1	8.5
Merck (US)	44.0	7.5	9.5	4.4
GSK (UK)	41.4	5.3	9.9	8.5
AstraZeneca (UK)	25.7	4.3	7.3	12.6

Source: GlobalData
(http://www.bbc.co.uk/news/business-28212223)

Before you read on, just take a minute to stop and *really* look at Figure 3.1…These drug companies are making an absolute fortune! The revenues of many of these global businesses are greater than the gross domestic product (GDP) of entire countries. Also have a look at the research and development

(R&D) spent in comparison to revenue. These drug companies try to justify the cost of their medication because the cost of testing and researching drugs is so enormous. That's true – it is. But when those same companies can legally suppress clinical trial data and cherry-pick the results that suit their objective – to get the drug approved so they can sell it – then the clinical trials are actually a farce (see the Reboxetine example below). Which means that we (personally, our medical insurance company or the NHS) are buying incredibly expensive drugs that may not even work for us, may actually make us sicker or – worse – kill us. In fact, in his book *Deadly Psychiatry and Organised Denial*, author Professor Peter Gøtzsche states that the third highest cause of death in the UK after heart disease and cancer is psychiatric drugs! And Gøtzsche should know – he's an investigator for the independent Cochrane Collaboration – an international body that assesses medical research. Considering that 80 million prescriptions for psychiatric drugs are written in the UK alone every year that's terrifying.

The purpose of many of these drugs is clearly not about health and well-being, it's about money, money and more money. For example, some cancer drugs cost upwards of $100,000 for a full course. But they cost a fraction of that to manufacture. How much incentive is there for pharmaceutical companies to find a cure for cancer when they can make that sort of money treating it? In 2013 100 leading oncologists from around the world wrote an open letter in the journal *Blood* calling for a reduction in the price of cancer drugs. Dr Brian Druker, director of the Knight Cancer Institute, and one of the signatories, asked: 'If you are making $3bn a year on Gleevec [a cancer drug], could you get by with $2bn? When do you cross the line from essential profits to profiteering?'

But that's not all. Look at the sales and marketing spend in comparison to the R & D spend. In some cases it's almost double. So hang on, drug companies say they charge so much and profit from other people's misery because the cost of R & D is so huge – only the R & D is a lie and actually the companies spend twice that trying to convince us – patients and doctors – that it's not.

Oh, and by the way, sales and marketing for big pharmaceutical companies is not about where to place a full-page advertisement in what national newspaper or what TV commercial to make. It's actually lobbying health groups to lower 'the healthy limit' to create new markets like the cholesterol example I shared in the last chapter, or seeking approval to market the drug to a different demographic, or rebranding the same drug for a different condition. Often this approach ends in fines. For example, GlaxoSmithKline were fined $3 billion in 2012 for promoting Paxil for depression to under-18-year-olds. In 2009, Pfizer was fined $2.3 billion over misbranding the painkiller Bextra. Johnson & Johnson was fined $2.2 billion in 2013 for promoting drugs not approved as safe. In 2012 Abbott was fined $1.5 billion for illegal promotion of the antipsychotic drug Depakote. Eli Lilly were in trouble in 2009 and fined $1.4 billion for wrongly promoting antipsychotic drug Zyprexa and Merck was fined $950 million in 2011 for illegally promoting painkiller Vioxx.

These are huge fines but they are nothing to the money that was made before the fine was imposed. Plus these companies have epic legal teams fighting these battles every day. Even when they are fined these faceless corporations are still the winners, as evidenced by their billion-dollar revenues year on year.

The other really popular sales and marketing tactic is to create new 'conditions'. I have a friend who ran a half-marathon in Sydney a few years ago and she ended up running with a PR officer for a large pharmaceutical company. She had actually just quit her job because she couldn't stand it any more – most of her job involved sitting around the corporate boardroom with other sales and marketing executives dreaming up new diseases, disorders or conditions that the team could then publicise and sell products for. This practice is so morally and ethically screwed up that it's hard to believe it actually happens and yet it is normal business practice in big pharmaceutical companies.

And of course we've lapped it up…We have become obsessed

with health and we are increasingly conscious of when we don't feel well. So we 'Google' our symptoms and before lunchtime we have shortlisted our disease to two pages of A4 paper. Come on, admit it – you've done it. We've all done it! We could easily mount a very strong case, especially in the developed Western world, that we are a bunch of hypochondriacs. But the drug companies have had a direct hand in creating our collective hypochondria. As a sales and marketing strategy it's pure genius – dream up new 'conditions', advertise the condition to raise our awareness of it, so we can think we have it and then sell us the cure!

It's just a lie based on money and it rarely has anything to do with you or your health.

Ever since antibiotics the scientific community and the big pharmaceutical companies have sought to find a magic bullet that will cure every condition on the planet. This objective was brought ever closer once the human genome was mapped. Today there are hundreds of thousands of scientists around the world trying to isolate what gene causes what condition so pharmaceutical companies can patent it and sell us the drug for ever. Of course, it's not yet yielded the fruits they were hoping for because human beings are incredibly complex and what works for one will not necessarily work for another. The way our genes express themselves depends on a myriad of factors, from diet to environment, to physiology to gender, to ethnicity and beyond. So the very idea that we will reach a point where one pill will cure cancer, diabetes, obesity etc. is almost science fiction.

Please understand, I'm a huge fan of science and the people on the front line doing the research and genuinely seeking cures for terrible conditions, but I am not a fan of the companies that are so often pulling the strings or funding that research (often without the researchers knowing about it) so they can profit from illness and misery.

According to a recent global analysis project, if current trends continue, depression will be the second greatest disease burden by the year 2020 and the first by 2030. It is now estimated that 350 million people globally are affected by depression. And that doesn't take other mental health issues into account.

Mental health is booming. Not just in terms of the escalating number of drugs created to 'treat it' but the escalating number of mental health disorders to treat. In the last 20 years there has been a huge increase in the number of new 'mental health disorders' classified and labelled. People who were previously viewed as simply shy, eccentric, or easily bored are now labelled with a disorder or condition. *The Diagnostic and Statistical Manual of Mental Disorders (DSM)* – the 'go-to guide' for all mental illness – adds new entries to their book every year, voted in by a show of hands in a room full of men in suits. Last year they even added 'Internet gaming disorder' to their list of mental health disorders and have requested further study to decide which medication is best to prescribe. Again, this is not about health and well-being. This is about money. If something can be labelled, then big pharmaceutical companies can sell pills to medicate it!

And, with such huge numbers lining up to take those pills (often for non-existent conditions) it's easy to see why, in 2015, the mental health pharmaceutical market was estimated to be worth \$88.3 billion. And of course, once someone is prescribed antidepressants, many of which are very addictive, that revenue is going to pour in for years, possibly decades.

I suppose in some ways we should be grateful – before Thorazine (the brand name for chlorpromazine) was developed in the 1950s mental illness was often treated with surgery – known as a lobotomy. In fact, the man who developed this psychosurgery procedure was awarded the Nobel Prize for his work in 1949. When a patient had a lobotomy the surgeon removed part of the brain. Now considering that in 2016 we still don't yet know all the mysteries of the brain and probably know more about the surface of the moon than we do about the interconnections and functions of the human brain, slicing off chunks doesn't seem like a particularly sophisticated approach. And yet unbelievably, more than 20,000 people underwent lobotomies in the US during the 1940s until these new drugs were invented to treat our madness.

My Early Experiences of Madness Medication

I was first prescribed antidepressants in my late teens and, to be honest, I didn't notice much difference in the first few weeks. In fact, I started to doubt whether they were working. But a week or so later, they kicked in and my world went from glorious Technicolor and the ups and downs of life to bland black and white. My feisty, sassy personality disappeared as I descended into the uneventful world of life on antidepressants. I don't know what it's like for you – but for me nothing seemed to matter that much any more. Things that I would normally get so worked up about would just breeze past without incident. I didn't get overly excited about anything but nor did I get overly upset by anything. I wasn't happy but I wasn't sad either and initially that stability was a relief. I was glad to be rid of the black dog that had burdened me for years – it was a welcome respite from feelings of self-loathing and hopelessness. I got used to the metallic taste in my mouth and the broken sleep at night. I hated the weight gain but at least I could function during the day without crying – so I kept taking the pills.

This went on for years until I fell pregnant and decided to stop – 'cold turkey'. For the record, cold turkey is not a good idea when stopping antidepressants. In hindsight, I think I was saved from severe withdrawal because there were so many happy hormones pumping around my body as a result of the pregnancy. Carrying my son was an epiphany. During the months he grew in my belly, I remember driving to work and the sky really did look bluer to me, my perception was heightened, I noticed more, I felt like a child again full of wonder and excitement for the future. I remember looking at the planes in the sky as I travelled to work, singing along to tunes on the radio and feeling the best I'd ever felt in my life! Of course, I put this down to the pregnancy hormones coursing through my body. It certainly didn't occur to me at the time that my new 'Ms Blue Sky' feelings may have been down to the fact that I was religiously taking folic acid and various vitamins and of course I was no longer taking the fluoxetine antidepressant. I was too busy enjoying the novelty of optimism – I felt alive for the first time in years and when my son was born I was on top of the world – despite a pretty horrific birth.

Unfortunately it didn't last. Once I'd stopped taking the supplements I'd been taking throughout my pregnancy things soon returned to my grim 'normal'. I panicked, looking after myself had been hard enough and now I had a beautiful newborn baby to look after, so I went back to the doctors. Of course, I was immediately put back on the antidepressants, along with a long lecture for coming off them in the first place. Within a matter of weeks

I was back to the old routine. I couldn't work out what was worse, the depression or the fact that I felt like I was back to square one.

Things were OK for a while, I seemed to be able to deal with everyday life, but then I suffered a bereavement and that tipped me over the edge into a full-on nosedive. My doctor increased my dose and that's when I really noticed a difference. It was like taking drugs in a nightclub except the music was scary and I was the only person on the dance floor with a spotlight on me. As a single parent I really struggled to cope, sitting in my living room on my own as my young son lay in bed, not knowing how I could care for him, or how I could face work in the morning. I was tripping out of my head but Pink Floyd wasn't playing in the background. I experienced hallucinations, terrors and thoughts most of us couldn't even imagine. It was horrific and even though I was in a mess I knew medication was not the answer. I went back to my doctor for help but he just put me on a different type of antidepressant (paroxetine).

Although I wasn't even sure, it was possible the new drug made things even worse. The black dog was back with a vengeance and this time I couldn't fend him off. I remember sitting crouched on my kitchen floor terrified of the future. I just didn't know what to do so I called my parents and I will never forget the confused look on their faces as they took my son – now a toddler – away to their house 'for safekeeping'.

I phoned in sick to work and spent days in bed. When I surfaced I started researching online for an alternative solution because the one I was prescribed was clearly not working. I discovered orthomolecular medicine – a form of alternative medicine which was based on maintaining health through nutritional supplementation and had men like Max Gerson, Abram Hoffer and Linus Pauling (the only man in history to have won the Nobel Prize twice) supporting its efficacy. In other words, these great scientists were coming out and publicly saying this approach really worked. Plus there was a whole bunch of studies and clinical evidence that supported the theories.

I thought if twice-winning Nobel laureates are promoting this stuff then there must be something in it – so I investigated further. There are days, I'm not even sure I'd still be here if I hadn't – it literally saved my life. And it absolutely changed my life! And my son's too. He had been suffering from chronic food allergies, asthma and eczema, and the doctors had prescribed steroid ointments, Ventolin syrup and inhalers. When he was just four years old he nearly died on a holiday when he had an allergic reaction to a pony he was riding in the mountains. He had an almost immediate reaction to the pony and his face blew up like a balloon and he could hardly speak. Unbelievably, a Canadian lady who was also on the tour had a bottle of Benadryl in her handbag, she pushed his tongue, which was now huge, to the side and poured it down his throat. The antihistamine in the Benadryl was enough to stop the swelling from getting any worse while I drove like a maniac to get him to hospital for a steroid injection. If that lady hadn't had a cold and hadn't had the Benadryl in her bag my son would probably have died. In a separate incident I had to take him to hospital in Chicago after he ate some chocolate pudding.

Thankfully, I immersed myself in orthomolecular medicine and we changed our diet and started to take supplements. Within a matter of months my son's allergies miraculously disappeared, he could breathe without the need of an inhaler, and I lowered my dose of antidepressants one week at a time until I was finally free of them 12 weeks later. I'll explain exactly how I achieved this in the action plan later in the book, so you can see if you can successfully and safely do the same.

Other than the odd podiatrist appointment due to an ingrown toenail, my son and I have not visited the doctor in almost a decade. Touch wood – we never get the flus, colds and stomach bugs that everyone else seems to get and we are both fighting fit!

Turning Back the Clock

Before big pharmaceutical companies muscled in to profit from our madness and ill health, early pioneers intent on finding answers, not money-making opportunities, were doing amazing and important work.

In the early 1900s, for example, psychiatrists like the infamous Dr Henry Cotton practised experimental 'surgical bacteriology' on mental health patients. The thinking at the time was that insanity was the result of untreated infections. Dr Cotton would remove teeth and various organs from patients in an effort to rid the body of infection. The colon was of particular interest and doctors believed that bad bacteria in the gut, or as they called it at the time 'intestinal putrefaction', was the cause of mental illness. Therefore if the doctor removed the colon or part of the colon then the patient would be restored to normal health. The main stumbling block to this theory was that antibiotics had not yet been invented, so the surgery ended up killing one in three patients.

However, other doctors at the time such as Doctors Louis Julianelle and Franklin G. Ebaugh discovered a less invasive method of treating patients, stating, 'We do not believe that colectomy is justifiable. Putrefaction, if present, may be eliminated by a change in the intestinal flora.'

Their paper, 'Implantation of Bacillus and Acidophilus in Persons with Psychoses', published in 1923 was a study based on treating mental health patients by populating their guts with good bacteria. It never ceases to amaze me just how ironic it is that despite our breakthroughs and innovations we have repeatedly turned our back on common sense that our grandparents seemed to already know, not to mention the insightful science and accurate diagnosis in favour of the flashy answer or the magic potion. And we are still doing it today.

It has taken a while but finally, some 100 years later, scientists are now recognising the link between good bacteria in the gut and mental health. You simply can't have one without the other.

Doctors in the Dark

I'm sure, like me, you rely on your doctor and you may already be thinking, 'OK, but hang on. Surely if all this were true our doctor would know about it and they would be making alternative suggestions.' It's a perfectly reasonable question and the answer is that doctors should know about this but they don't. But before you get upset at your doctor – it's often not their fault.

There are a number of issues that keep doctors in the dark about the importance of nutrition and especially the key role of micronutrients in the diet and how their loss can have a profound impact on our mental and physical well-being.

The first is that they are simply not taught about it in medical school. In the mid 1980s, a landmark report by the *National Academy of Sciences* highlighted the lack of adequate nutrition education in medical schools and the writers recommended a minimum of 25 hours of nutrition instruction. Two and a half decades later, a 2010 study by researchers at the University of North Carolina, Chapel Hill, found that the vast majority of medical schools still fail to meet the minimum recommended 25 hours of instruction. Only a quarter of 100 medical schools surveyed offered the recommended 25 hours on nutrition – four schools offered nutrition as an option, and one school offered nothing at all.

But even at 25 hours, it's nowhere near enough time to understand the impact of nutrition on the body. It isn't close to adequate for doctors to understand the various minerals, vitamins and micronutrients we need in the body and how a lack of one can have a knock-on effect elsewhere. The human body is a highly interconnected, subtle and extremely complex system, and yet we know virtually nothing about the fuel we put into the system and how it can impact performance. You wouldn't buy a Ferrari and put fizzy juice in it and expect to get very far, and yet we have an amazing body and we constantly put crap in it and expect to live long and healthy lives.

To be fair to doctors, results of a study carried out in the Aberdeen district of Scotland showed that despite their ignorance on the subject, over 90 per cent of doctors requested more teaching on the practical aspects of nutrition. Indeed both medical students and junior doctors were very enthusiastic to learn about nutrition, and also felt that their teaching was inadequate.

The other big issue that keeps doctors in the dark is time.

Just think about everything that a GP needs to know. It's a genuinely phenomenal amount. But even once they qualify and start practising they also have to keep up to date with latest breakthroughs. Those that specialise become an 'ologist' of one form or another and tend to have a deeper and deeper knowledge about a narrower and narrower field. Often those fields have their own language and argue over finer and finer points of differentiation, which means that getting up to date and staying up to date is almost impossible. Plus doctors always have a waiting room of patients to attend to.

Even if they did manage to carve out some time to research the latest drugs on offer or the latest procedures, they often don't have access to accurate clinical trials data when making decisions about what drugs to prescribe to patients.

Before a drug is approved for use the drug company has to invest billions in clinical trials – these are supposed to make sure the drug works and to find out about any side effects the medication may have. It would make sense therefore that doctors, or other medical professionals who could interpret that data, should have access to all the results of the various clinical trials. But that doesn't happen. What you may not know about clinical trials is that a drug company is under no legal obligation to share those results. So they only ever publish the data of the clinical trials that worked and bury the trials that didn't. So when your GP is punching in their diagnosis of your condition the recommended drugs that come back are often based on erroneous or incomplete clinical trial data. Neither you nor your doctor have any way of knowing whether you match the profile of people on the successful clinical trial, in which case the drug might work, or whether you fit the demographic of the clinical trials where the drug didn't work or, worse, created severe side effects.

Take the antidepressant Reboxetine as an example; Ben Goldacre writes about this in his brilliant book *Bad Pharma*. (If you want to get really mad – I highly recommend you read that book!) When he's not writing books that lift the lid on medicine he's a GP and he readily admits he has prescribed Reboxetine himself.

He'd looked at the available clinical trial data and considered them well-designed trials with overwhelmingly positive results. It was shown to be better than placebo and better than head-to-head comparisons with other antidepressants. And, it was approved by the Medicines and Healthcare products Regulatory Agency (MHRA) which governs all drugs in the UK. Millions of people around the world are on Reboxetine. In October 2010 a group of researchers managed to collect *all* the clinical trial data for *all* the trials of Reboxetine. The result was *very* different. Seven trials had been conducted comparing the drug with a placebo or sugar pill. Only one of those trials, with 254 patients, showed a positive result against a sugar pill with no pharmaceutical properties at all. Needless to say that trial was published in an academic journal for doctors and researchers to read. But it was publication bias, or at best an anomaly, caused by something other than the drug. How else can we explain the fact that the other six trials which featured almost ten times as many patients showed that Reboxetine was no better than the sugar pill? Of course, none of those trials were published anywhere.

So millions of people are being prescribed a drug that they believe is going to make them feel better when in actual fact they would be better off taking a jelly bean every day. But that's not the worst of it. It's blatant profiteering, but at least it's not doing any harm – right? Unbelievably no, that's not the case.

In other trials Reboxetine was compared to other antidepressant medication and 507 patients demonstrated that the drug did just as well in head-to-head tests. Again that trial was published. *Again* doctors and researchers, like Ben Goldacre, would read these results and be further convinced of the efficacy of the new drug. Many, like Ben Goldacre, probably went on to prescribe Reboxetine as a result. But there were another 1,657 patients who took the new drug and they all did worse than those on other drugs. Again, that data was squirrelled away and not published anywhere. But it gets worse.

In terms of side effects Reboxetine looked fine in all the published papers about the drug that appeared in academic and medical journals. But when the researchers looked at all the clinical trial data it turned out that patients were more likely to have side effects – and were more likely to stop taking the drug and withdraw from the trial because of those side effects than when they took the comparison drugs. As Goldacre states, 'In the published data, Reboxetine was a safe and effective drug. In reality, it was no better than a sugar pill and, worse, it does more harm than good.'

What you absolutely have to understand is this is not a one-off isolated incident or event – this is business as usual in big pharmaceutical companies and it's not limited to this one drug. In fact it's almost unfair to call out Reboxetine because it implies this is rare. It's not rare – what is rare is that researchers were able to get access to all the clinical trials. That is almost impossible.

Even though the World Health Organization (WHO) made a fresh call for the public disclosure of all clinical trial data in 2015, there is so far no change to the law and no change to 'business as usual' for the big pharmaceutical companies.

The drug companies are of course resisting – very strongly. For a start many of the drugs simply wouldn't get approved if all the data was available. Plus many of these clinical trials also include placebo trials – many of which demonstrate that a sugar pill or saline injection delivered by a doctor is just as effective as the drug company's expensive new drug. At the moment these results are also suppressed. After all, even drug companies can't charge billions of dollars for Smarties!

The same thing has happened in complementary and herbal medicine. Despite the fact that herbs have well-documented healing powers that have been used by human beings for thousands of years, in 2002 the EU and UK tried to ban vitamins and herbal remedies. Luckily there was a public outcry, but in 2011 EU rules came into force banning hundreds of herbal remedies – forcing many natural practitioners and manufacturers out of business. As a result, in the UK today herbal remedies – medicines and treatment that have been used successfully for millennia – have to be assessed by the Medical and Healthcare products Regulatory Agency (MHRA) and are only allowed to go on sale to the public if the MHRA approve them. This is in stark contrast to the downright dangerous drugs that are already on sale by big pharmaceutical companies based on incomplete clinical trial data. Something is seriously wrong when GPs regularly hand out antidepressants with thousands of side effects – some of them lethal – but the notion of taking plants as medicine is somehow more dangerous? It's utterly ludicrous.

In the UK herbal remedies now need to be registered on the Traditional Herbal Registration (THR) scheme – a process which costs many thousands of pounds for each remedy. This has all but crippled small independent herbalists who don't have the means to register their products – often remedies they have used safely and effectively for years. The THR scheme can also only be used for minor ailments – not chronic conditions – further stifling the industry. Of course, this government intervention, usually aided by big business lobbying, plays right into the hands of the pharmaceutical companies because their natural remedy competitors have to either increase the price to cover the costs of registration or they simply go out of business altogether. This is why herbal medicines are so expensive compared to over-the-counter pharmaceutical drugs.

Plus if you look on the UK NHS website, for example, you will find some terrifying information about herbal medicine. Visitors are warned, 'You may experience a bad reaction', and 'They may cause problems if you are taking other medicines'. 'Pregnant women, breastfeeding mothers, children and the elderly should avoid them', 'Using them for more serious conditions could put you at risk'. We are told, 'The claims made for herbal medicines are based on traditional usage and not on evidence of the products' effectiveness.' Claims made by big pharmaceutical companies are often not even based on traditional use and, in many cases, little evidence of the products' effectiveness, and yet they are sold in their billions, often with serious and extremely dangerous side effects.

Clearly there are some pharmaceutical drugs that have been immensely important for human health but it doesn't alter the fact that we've used plants since the beginning of human history to heal ourselves and thousands of studies show they're effective. The scaremongering by those who want to sell us something else instead is all about money and control, and nothing about health and well-being.

It's also bonkers when you consider there are 4,719 evidence-based herbal medicine research paper links on the National Institute for Health and Care Excellence (NICE) website – an organisation and website that is part of the UK government Department of Health. Talk about mixed messages! Of course, those looking for advice on herbal medicine are unlikely to find that website. Instead they will probably log on to the NHS site for information – information that is likely to scare them away from herbal medicine or any complementary medicine techniques and approaches.

What you have to remember is that the goal of big pharmaceutical companies is not health – it's money. In the same way that food companies continuously sell us diet products that don't work but give us hope, drug companies are happy to continuously sell us drugs that don't work but give us hope. Often they are making a huge amount of money by simply masking the symptoms or treating the condition and are not even genuinely looking for a cure. And they don't want placebos, herbal or complementary medicine screwing with their profits so they seek to discredit the alternatives instead.

Finally, the last, although connected, issue that is keeping doctors in the dark is a combination of the other two. Doctors don't have enough time to do the research so they rely on others to keep them abreast of new drugs and developments. Often those 'others' are pharmaceutical company sales reps. The doctors are therefore being 'informed' by the very people charged with selling the resulting drugs to GPs so they will prescribe them to their patients and boost profits. You don't need to be Einstein to realise that this 'information' is seriously biased.

NHS cardiologist Dr Aseem Malhotra, the doctor leading the call for a public inquiry into drug companies' 'murky' practices, warned that commercial conflicts of interest are contributing to an 'epidemic of misinformed doctors and misinformed patients in the UK and beyond'. Dr Malhotra stated, 'There is no doubt that a "more medicine is better" culture lies at the heart of healthcare, exacerbated by financial incentives within the system to prescribe more drugs and carry out more procedures. But there's a more sinister barrier to making progress to raise awareness of – and thus tackle – such issues that we should be most concerned about, and that's the information that is being provided to doctors and patients to guide treatment decisions.' Dr Malhotra accused drug companies of 'gaming the system' by spending twice as much on marketing than on research. Something I drew your attention to earlier in this chapter.

Wrap Up

I have come to believe that almost all mental illnesses – apart from the criminally insane – can be cured with love and a good diet. This is not a novel opinion. Hippocrates, the father of medicine and the man who created the Hippocratic oath, taken by doctors to 'first, do no harm', mostly prescribed food, herbs and sometimes wine to his patients. There's always a silver lining!

The link between nutrition and mental health is undeniable and one that must be taken seriously by GPs and psychiatrists before scribbling that prescription for psychotropic drugs. The drugs on their own won't cure you and can even hinder recovery as you then have the problem of coming off them. Plus in many cases they can make things worse because they are packed with ingredients that further damage our brain and body.

In a comprehensive peer-reviewed paper published in the *International Journal of Health and Nutrition* in 2013, the authors cited over 100 research studies in support of their evaluation that lack of certain nutrients can contribute to the formation of psychiatric disease and we will fully explain which ones and why in the following pages.

This is great news for everyone who is currently fat, mad or both, because it means that we can eradicate the mad fat epidemic. We can heal ourselves and it's time to learn how.

Part Three
Get Educated

'Insanity: doing the same thing over and over again and expecting different results.'

– Albert Einstein

Chapter 4: Time to Get Angry

'Advertising is legalised lying.'

– H. G. Wells

Before we dive into the action plan so you can heal yourself, there are a few other things you need to be aware of.

First of all, I really hope that you *are* mad! Not the type of mad that doctors want to prescribe a pill for, but rather the hopping up and down with rage sort of mad. You should be and you have every right to be. We are being lied to. We are given false information touted as 'fact' and we are being manipulated into buying food and other products that are often making us sick – physically and mentally. And this has been going on for decades.

You may not have heard of a man called Edward Bernays but he is widely considered the father of public relations. Bernays was the American nephew of famous psychoanalyst Sigmund Freud and, although relatively unknown, his influence on the twentieth century is every bit as profound as his famous uncle.

By any standard, Freud's theories range from the valid, to the interesting, to the downright bizarre. Much of his work was focused on hidden forces in the human psyche that needed to be controlled otherwise it could lead individuals and societies to chaos and destruction. Remember this was a time when the average person didn't really have much say in their life, but that was changing. Those in power didn't like the implications so they attempted to use Freud's theories to control the crowd and therefore hang on to the power.

Bernays was the first person to take Freud's ideas about human beings and use them to manipulate the masses. For the first time, he was able to show US companies how they could make people want things they didn't need by linking mass-produced goods to their unconscious desires.

Bernays had appreciated the potential of Freud's ideas but – perhaps more importantly – had seen their impact first-hand. As the US announced they were entering the First World War it set up a committee on public information and Bernays was employed to promote the US war aims in the press. US president at the time Woodrow Wilson declared that US involvement was not about restoring the old empires but to bring democracy to all of Europe. Bernays proved very skilful at promoting this idea in the US and abroad. So much so that he was invited to join President Wilson at the Paris peace talks after the war. It was in Paris that he realised just how effective his art for propaganda really was. President Wilson was welcomed as a hero and liberator of the masses, and as Bernays watched the crowds surge around the president he wondered if it would be possible to achieve the same type of mass persuasion to get people to buy products. Bernays is even on record as saying, 'When I came back to the United States I decided that if you could use propaganda for war, you could certainly use it for peace.' And use it he did – although he changed the name of what he did from 'propaganda' to 'public relations' to avoid the negative implications 'propaganda' still has today.

Bernays was sure he could influence human behaviour, especially buying behaviour, if he could tap into people's unconscious, irrational desires and emotions. He realised that there was a lot more going on in human decision-making than logical information. We know this – right? We know that having that third can of fizzy juice and another takeaway dinner isn't going to help how we feel but we do it anyway. We know we should get off the couch and go for a walk but the pull of the TV and a comforting snack after a long day at the office is much more emotionally appealing. So, we don't do it – even though we *know* we should.

One of Bernays's best-known peacetime propaganda

campaigns was called 'Torches of Freedom', to promote smoking to women. By the 1920s, tobacco companies were doing a roaring trade selling cigarettes to men but it was still considered taboo for women to smoke, especially in public. Imagine the possibilities though – just by somehow breaking that taboo, the cigarette companies could immediately *double* their market. So American Tobacco Company hired Bernays to do just that. Using psychoanalysis made famous by his uncle, Bernays discovered that, to women, cigarettes were seen as a symbol of male domination. He believed that if he could reposition smoking as a challenge to that perceived male power, tapping into women's desire for more freedom, then they would take to smoking like ducks to water. To test the theory he persuaded a group of rich, beautiful debutantes to hide cigarettes under their clothes and join the Easter Day parade in New York. Bernays would give the women a signal and they were to light up the cigarettes in public. At the same time Bernays informed the press that a group of suffragettes were planning to use the Easter Day parade to protest by lighting up their 'Torches of Freedom'.

So when the ladies fired up their cigarettes at the parade the press were already there in huge numbers to capture the moment for their respective newspapers. On 1 April 1929 *The New York Times* printed: 'Group of Girls Puff at Cigarettes as a Gesture of "Freedom"'. Almost overnight, smoking became a symbol of emancipation for women and the image helped to break the taboo that prevented women from smoking in public.

Effectively millions of women were manipulated into smoking. Smoking is extremely bad for your health. Granted, we've only proven that categorically since the 1950s, so perhaps Bernays did see his campaign as a way towards equal rights for women, but it's highly doubtful. Regardless of his true motives, his masterful propaganda repositioned smoking for women as an act of liberation and freedom of expression, and he did it in order to sell more cigarettes. Slogans such as 'An ancient prejudice has been removed' (Lucky Strike) or 'You've come a long way, baby' (Virginia Slims) appealed to women's hopes and dreams for greater freedom and equality. Bernays himself said breaking down the barriers to women smoking was 'like opening a new gold mine right in American Tobacco's front yard'.

We are being manipulated by smart people who understand what buttons they need to press to get us to buy certain products – and keep buying them. Only sometimes, like with cigarettes, those products are actively killing us! But it's not just cigarettes – this problem is rife in modern food production where we are constantly being hoodwinked into believing certain products are healthy when they're not.

Slick Marketing and Widespread Manipulation

There are thousands, probably hundreds of thousands, of people like Edward Bernays plying their trade in big food or retail marketing departments all over the world. There are whole fields of research, including behavioural economics and social science, that explores why we do what we do so companies can exploit that information and make us buy more.

This means that the chips (excuse the pun) are seriously stacked against us.

When we go out to the supermarket, to a restaurant, to the cinema – or anywhere else where we'll be faced with food choices – we need to think more like Lara Croft and less like Pac-Man. Are we mindless yellow blobs programmed to consume everything that crosses our path – or are we sentient, empowered women, who don't let other people tell us what to do? (Of course, you've probably just realised I've also just used Bernays's technique to push your emotional buttons. No one wants to be a 'mindless yellow blob' but most of us would be quite happy to associate ourselves with the kick-ass character played by Angelina Jolie!)

The point you need to appreciate is that it's a war out there and we must be prepared for battle. There are three levels of manipulation you need to be aware of. First are the sounds, smells and bright signage enticing you to buy and eat something which your body doesn't need and isn't feeding your brain. The next level is the awkward upsell from the cute guy at the checkout – 'Would you like fries with that?' or 'Can I tempt you with one of our chocolate bar offers today?' We experience these upsells whether we are buying stamps in the post office, the weekly shop in the supermarket, or even the chemist! Even if we've stayed strong we then usually need to watch other people scoffing the very thing we fought so hard to avoid!

If we want to win the game we need to be like Lara Croft. No messing. No negotiating. We simply must focus on the end goal – improved health and mental well-being. Of course, everyone trying to sell you their products wants you to behave like Pac-Man – gobbling up everything they offer and still looking for more.

Next time you are in a shop look at the difference in product marketing in different categories. How many smiley faces, bright-coloured packaging, alluring language and money-off specials do you see in the fresh produce aisle compared to, say, cereals, soft drinks and confectionery? It is usually boxes of high-fat snacks, sugar-laden drinks or sugar-coated cereals that are piled up on shelf-end gondolas or at the front of the store under big colourful banners. We are reminded of just how much money we can save if we buy enough to feed a small army. Retailers know we are suckers for a bargain and will use every trick in the book to get us to buy more than we actually need. The buy one, get one free offers, or BOGOF offers as they are called in the industry, are very popular in supermarkets. As are 50 per cent extra free, half price, extra points on your loyalty card, win a prize, get a cuddly toy, etc. If you look closely most of these discounts and offers are on processed foods, fake food or sugar-laden food with high profit margins. Certainly, I've yet to see a crate of apples or box of broccoli marketed in bulk at such discounted prices. There is a reason for that – money. Getting you to part with yours for food that makes you fat and miserable! Seriously – it's a terrible trade. Get smart. Don't be fooled. Learn to beat the retailers and big food processors at their own game.

Easy Step: If you have a fat or mad friend, go shopping together. That way you can support each other to avoid those tempting offers. And if you do succumb you can split the BOGOF offers so you save money and buy less.

Make it into a game. I do this with my son when we are shopping or even when we are watching the news. Instead of telling him about the countless ways we are being manipulated to feel a certain way about a news story, or feel a certain way about a product so we buy it, I ask him questions about what he actually sees. Sometimes it's hilarious because once you start to notice this blatant manipulation it's almost comical. And once we see it for what it is, it starts to lose its subconscious power to direct our behaviour and alter our mood.

Use of colour

Colour is one of the weapons of choice in food marketing and it's used in a variety of ways to influence what we buy and how much we consume. Colour psychology studies show that certain colours are more likely to make us feel agitated, while other colours have a calming, soothing effect.

The primary red and yellow colours frequently used at fast-food outlets are carefully chosen to get us in and out of the establishment as quickly as possible. Companies like McDonald's, KFC and Burger King are volume-driven businesses and want you to 'grab and go' so they can serve more customers and make more money. Most of us can eat a Big Mac meal with a chocolate milkshake in just over five minutes, consuming our daily allowance of calories in the blink of an eye. These fast-food giants don't want us to hang around; they don't want us to question the nutritional value or source of the food they serve. Instead, they rely on the instant gratification approach to eating, where we have no time to consider the fat we've just lathered on our hips or the sugar poisoning our brains.

The colour of their outdoor signage is no accident either – red has the longest wavelength, it triggers stimulation, appetite and feelings of hunger. Yellow triggers feelings of happiness and friendliness due to its association with the sun. It also attracts attention – yellow is the most visible colour in daylight and, as any parent will tell you, McDonald's golden arches seem to be visible to children from miles away! Interestingly, McDonald's are now changing the colours of many of their outlets in affluent areas where they are struggling to compete with the premium burger chains and coffee shops. Their new green livery elicits feelings of nature, as they battle to capture more affluent consumers that are interested in animal welfare, sustainability and prefer more natural products.

At the other end of the market, 'white tablecloth' restaurants want you to stick around – to splash out on their extensive dessert menu, maybe enjoy a cheeky wee Irish coffee, a liqueur, or another bottle of their ridiculously overpriced wine. Upscale eateries use soft tones, natural browns and green colours, along with mood lighting and soft music to encourage customers to relax, take their time and enjoy the *experience* as well as the food and drink.

Colours on food packaging have been carefully chosen too. Black, metallic colours, burgundy reds, royal blues and deep dark colours signify premium and are often used in aspirational brands to signify quality (whether or not the product is quality or not). Blues are most often used for so-called 'health' foods or diet products – whether they are or not. And browns and greens signify natural, wholesome or organic products – whether they are or not! And we fall for it – hook, line and sinker.

Big food companies have been controlling our behaviour and manipulating our buying behaviour for decades and they often know what we are going to buy before we do. The language of colour is communicated quicker to the brain than words or shapes and work directly on our feelings and emotions. Basically food producers and retailers are hijacking our brain to trigger emotions that make us reach for their products and put them in our basket.

It is perfectly legal but it's morally questionable at best and downright irresponsible at worst – especially when many of these foods have zero nutritional value and are not helping us battle the bulge or improve our mental well-being. It never ceases to amaze me that we get upset at the state of the nation's health – escalating consumption of alcohol, escalating diabetes and obesity and even a recognition of the escalating problem of mental health – but nothing changes. The government – whatever political persuasion – comes out with some new initiative or other but no one is actually tackling the cause: the products that are causing the problem. These outcomes are hardly a surprise when you can buy alcohol and fizzy drinks cheaper than milk or water in the local supermarket, when processed food is quick, convenient and often reasonably cheap, and when just about everything we buy is laden with sugar, preservatives and unpronounceable additives! It's time we wise up and we need to train our brains to override the subliminal 'buy me' programming. Just by being aware that this is happening to us can massively reduce the emotional pull food marketers have over our behaviour. It's easy to get conned when you don't know it's happening – it's much harder when you can see it for what it is.

> ***Easy Step:*** Next time you are in the supermarket take a look at the signage and positioning of products. What foods stand out? What signage draws your attention? What foods are on special offer? Where are the BOGOF deals? Take a moment to pick up some of those products and take a close look at the ingredients – how many are there? How many can you pronounce? We are being manipulated to pick those products up and put them in our basket without thinking. The question is are you happy to be the 'mindless yellow blob' or are you going to be 'Lara Croft'?

Change the Way You Look at Food

There is an old saying 'your eyes are bigger than your belly'. It's usually used by parents when their child has piled their plate with food and then can't finish it all. It's also true. Most of us need to reduce our portion sizes.

Studies show that children and adults eat more food when larger portions are served regardless of how hungry they are. A BBC One documentary called *Tomorrow's Food* hosted by Dara Ó Briain explored technology where the person would eat while wearing virtual reality goggles – they would see their own hand which would reach out and pick up the food and then eat it. In the first experiment Dr Shini Somara was asked to eat as many Oreo cookies as she could. Despite being a very slim TV presenter she managed an impressive eight. The next day she repeated the experiment but could only manage five and looked quite ill after the fifth. So what was the difference? Unknown to her the researchers had increased the virtual size of the cookie. Although Dr Shini asked several times if the cookies were bigger in the second experiment, they were the exact same Oreo brand she had eaten the day before. They just looked bigger on her virtual reality screen so her brain was tricked into believing they were bigger and so told her she was full much earlier.

I've tried this trick myself – albeit without the virtual reality goggles. If I have an early morning start following a big night in with the girls and don't have the time or inclination to nurse a hangover, I just use smaller glasses. Most of the time we don't even realise and still have an enjoyable night while drinking much less wine!

Easy Step: If you go to the cinema with your mad fat friends, ask for a couple of empty drinks' cups when you buy the popcorn and split the bucket of popcorn between your friends. Munching through a whole bucket each is mainly habit – this way you save money and still get the popcorn experience. Little tricks and tips like this, and reducing the size of wine glasses, can help trick our brains into eating and drinking less.

Easy Step: Don't be tempted to get the next size up just because it's a few pennies more – it might seem like a good deal for our wallets but it is doing our bellies and our brains no good at all!

People also eat the foods that are most easily available to them. A research team at Cornell University conducted a consumption experiment in the workplace. They placed bowls of M&M's at different parts of the office – some on the desks, some next to printers. When researchers counted up the number of M&M's eaten every night it was the bowl on the desks, in easy reach, that were usually empty. The point being, if you have food at your fingertips and don't have to make much effort to go and get it, you are far more likely to consume more.

Another thing to watch out for is something called 'sensory-specific satiety'. This is when a variety of food leads to increased consumption. In another Cornell-conducted M&M's study, researchers distributed bowls of M&M's – some with a variety of colours and some with just one colour. Of course, the M&M's aficionados among us already know that all M&M's taste the same, regardless of the colour of the outer shell. Unfortunately our brain doesn't really know that and reacts in strange yet predictable ways when presented with choice and variety. The Cornell study showed that bowls of different-coloured M&M's were consumed faster than the ones with just one colour. Our brain gets bored when eating the same flavour and neural connections signal to stop eating. However, when a new flavour is introduced the brain gets fired up again and signals to keep on eating. The interesting thing with the M&M's study is that the colour was the only difference and yet this was enough to trick the brain into thinking 'yummy – this is something new – let's eat more'.

This explains why we always eat more in 'all-you-can-eat' buffet restaurants or the 'Sunday carvery' where we get to choose a little roast beef, roast lamb, turkey, meat loaf, pork and just a wee sliver of chicken or ham, not to mention the potatoes cooked three ways, umpteen vegetables and condiments. This also explains why most boxes of chocolates contain different-flavoured sweets in different shapes with different-coloured wrappers. Food marketing gurus are well aware of this colour trickery too – that's why certain cereal brands – like Cheerios – have different-coloured hoops or children's confectionery brands like Haribo have different-shaped and coloured sweets which look different but taste the same. It has all been carefully studied and calculated to trick us into eating more and therefore buying more.

We absolutely must learn to look beyond the label and appreciate that we are being manipulated by clever advertisers who deliberately use psychological 'hot buttons'. All these companies care about is how to sell more products – they certainly don't care whether these products are contributing to the mad fat epidemic.

Chapter 5: Bad Halogens

'There is growing evidence that Americans would have better health and a lower incidence of cancer and fibrocystic disease of the breast if they consumed more iodine. A decrease in iodine intake coupled with an increased consumption of competing halogens, fluoride and bromide, has created an epidemic of iodine deficiency in America.'

– Dr Donald Miller Jr

Before we cover the various food groups and get into the action plan, we also need to understand that our challenge is not just down to the food we eat – whether we are mad, fat or both. There are also significant environmental concerns that we need to be aware of and manage. The biggest of which are bad halogens.

Bad halogens are fluoride, chlorine and bromine and they are in everything from our drinking water, food, washing powder, toothpaste, personal care products and cosmetics – even our clothes and household furnishings contain bad halogens. They are bad because they displace iodine (a good halogen) in the body. Iodine is essential for thyroid health and it is extremely important for regulating metabolism. A healthy metabolism is, of course, crucial for healthy weight. The problem is that iodine has a higher atomic weight (126.9 u) than any of the three bad halogens (fluorine is 18.99 u, chlorine is 35.45 u and bromine is 79.9 u) so can easily be displaced in the body. Think of fluoride, chlorine and bromine as halogen bullies that squash iodine. When there is an overabundance of the three bad halogens in the body they effectively neutralise the positive benefits of iodine. This can cause thyroid disruption, messing up hormone secretion and metabolism, which can create a whole host of health problems.

Considering that there are still parts of the world including the US, Ireland and parts of the UK where fluoride is added to the water supply this is very bad news, because fluoride displaces the positive benefits of iodine.

The thyroid, located in our neck, is one of the largest endocrine glands in the body. It is a very important gland because it controls how quickly we use energy, make proteins and control our sensitivity to other hormones. Part of its job is to take iodine from the blood and combine it with amino acids (the building blocks of protein) to form thyroid hormones. One of these hormones, thyroxine, is responsible for our metabolism which controls our weight. Our entire blood supply filters through our thyroid, extracting iodine, so it can do its job. If we are low on iodine, the thyroid cannot produce enough hormones, causing weight problems and mental illness.

Unfortunately, most people are deficient in the good halogen (iodine) and drowning in the bad halogens (fluoride, chlorine and bromine). In 2011 a study measuring iodine levels of 737 teenage girls was conducted at nine UK centres – Aberdeen, Belfast, Birmingham, Cardiff, Dundee, Exeter, Glasgow, London and Newcastle. Nearly 70 per cent of the samples revealed an iodine deficiency and almost a fifth (18 per cent) of samples showed very low iodine levels.

These low levels can lead to thyroid disorders and even people with mild thyroid disorders often have emotional or mental health symptoms as well as physical symptoms. Common emotional problems related to an overactive thyroid include anxiety, nervousness, butterflies in the stomach, racing heart, trembling, irritability and sleep difficulties. For those with an underactive thyroid, depression, low mood, tearfulness, loss of appetite and disturbed sleep are common. For both overactive and underactive thyroids, mood swings, short temper and insomnia are likely.

Other mental health problems with thyroid problems include: short-term memory lapses, lack of mental alertness and difficulties with concentration. Weight gain and difficulty losing weight is also a common complaint from women suffering from thyroid disorders.

In the 1950s a large body of research conducted in psychiatric hospitals revealed an association between hypothyroidism and depression. And guess what the most common cause of hypothyroidism is – yep, you guessed it…iodine deficiency. Studies have found that people with bipolar disorder also often have abnormal thyroid function.

Ironically, a few decades ago the populations of the US, Australia and the UK were not iodine deficient and yet today iodine levels are half what they were in the 1970s. Back then we got most of our iodine from fish, bread (containing iodised salt) and dairy products, but changes in our eating habits such as eating less fish and changes to food production have created widespread deficiency. There is, for example, no iodine added to bread any more, plus changes to the diet of dairy cattle has seen iodine levels in milk plummet. Children are also drinking less milk today – preferring fizzy drinks and sugary juices to the white stuff.

Salt is iodised in some countries, but government guidelines forcing processed food manufacturers to cut salt levels means we are consuming less iodine via salt. Of course, we have also been told that salt is bad for us which has further exacerbated the problem. The truth is too much salt *is* bad for us, but we still need iodine and if we are not getting it from iodised salt then where are we getting it from? It's ironic – the one thing we do seem to have cut back on – salt – is actually having an adverse knock-on effect because it's amplifying an already existing iodine deficiency that is contributing to our mad fat epidemic!

Easy Step: Instead of buying cheap table salt that does not contain iodine buy iodised salt. It's usually only a little more expensive but you need less of it and using it to season food helps you get enough iodine in your diet.

Fluoride

In March 2014 *The Lancet*, one of the most respected medical journals in the world, published a paper classifying fluoride as a neurotoxin, placing it in the same category as lead, arsenic, cyanide and mercury. In fact it's used as a rat poison. So why on earth are countries still adding it to drinking water? Ireland, the US, Australia, New Zealand and parts of the UK are some of these countries. It's utter madness.

What's especially ironic is that if we were not iodine deficient, iodine would help us to remove toxins from our body – including these extremely toxic heavy metals that fluoride has now been branded with!

According to Dr Robert Carlton PhD, former US Environmental Protection Agency (EPA) scientist, 'Fluoridation is the greatest case of scientific fraud of this century, if not all time.' And Dr Carlton is not alone; 14 Nobel Prize winners in chemistry and medicine now oppose the fluoridation of drinking water.

Of course, dentists tell us that fluoride prevents tooth decay and we must use it as preventative medicine – and no doubt they can cite a whole bunch of studies to support their claim. However, there was another dentist in the 1930s, Dr Weston Price, who joined the dots between nutrition and tooth decay. He studied Australian Aborigines, remote tribes in Africa, Canadian Indians and Eskimos where he found that isolated groups of people who were not eating a modern Western diet had *no* occurrence of tooth decay. Not a single case of tooth decay and yet there wasn't a toothbrush, mouthwash or tube of Colgate in sight . . . never mind a fluoridated water supply. These people were not eating processed 'industrial foods' but ate a diet far richer in minerals and vitamins than we do. You might be thinking, 'OK' but maybe that's down to their genetics'. But, that isn't the case because Dr Price also found that when these indigenous people started eating a Western diet they experienced the delights of tooth decay.

Besides, if adding fluoride to the drinking water is such a great idea to prevent tooth decay, why is it that around 90 per cent of people in the US still have tooth decay or experience it at some point in their lives? It's just another food myth pedalled by vested interests and those that simply don't know any better.

Easy Step: If you live in a country or area that adds fluoride to your drinking water then buy a water filter to remove as much as possible. In addition, try to find toothpaste that doesn't have fluoride in it – your local health food store should be able to help, or if you are feeling really adventurous try mixing coconut oil with a little bicarbonate of soda and make your own.

Chlorine

Chlorine is the second halogen bully. Its primary purpose is as a disinfectant. Again it is almost always added to drinking water as well as being a common disinfectant for swimming pools. In fact, a study published in *Pediatrics* in September 2009 showed that children who regularly swim in chlorinated swimming pools have increased risks of developing allergies or asthma. Adult swimmers have been linked with other health problems including bladder and rectal cancer.

Chlorine is also a neurotoxin. In fact it was chlorine that was used in the Second World War gas chambers. In nature chlorine exists as a chemical element and it is an essential mineral in our diet. However, industrial chlorine is not natural – it is produced by passing an electric current through ordinary salt (sodium chloride). The result is a poisonous gas which can then be used to form bleach, disinfectants, PVC piping, medicines, plastics and paints. It also kills people when they are exposed to large quantities in small areas such as Nazi gas chambers.

Unsurprisingly, this potent neurotoxin knocks out all bacteria – the good and the bad. This means that when ingested, chlorine kills all the bacteria in our guts including the microbes which help produce serotonin (our happy hormone). That killing power is what makes it so effective for disinfecting drinking water or swimming pools but it's pretty damaging for just about everything else. Needless to say, chlorine is an extremely harmful additive. Granted, it has its place but that place is nowhere near the human body – not in food, not in food processing and certainly not in our water. The water our ancestors drank from springs and mountains had natural chlorine in it – this is very different from the manufactured chemical muck many of us drink from our taps today.

A joint study conducted at the National Institute of Health Scientists and the University of Shizuoka in Japan found that natural organic substances react when exposed to chlorinated tap water and formed cancer-causing compounds named 'mutagen X' (MX), similar to well-known cancer-causing THMs (trihalomethanes). Another study conducted in Finland in 1997 showed that 'MX' is 170 times more deadly than other by-products of chlorination and the research showed damage to the thyroid gland.

Professor Carlson of the University of Minnesota, a strong opponent to water chlorination, said, 'The chlorine problem is similar to that of air pollution. Chlorine is the greatest crippler and killer of modern times.'

Easy Step: Again, if you live in an area where chlorine is added to your drinking water then use a filter. Ideally also add a filter to your shower head so you are less exposed to chlorine. Avoid chlorine-based cleaning products, but if you do use them, wear gloves to limit exposure to the skin. And stay away from some artificial sweeteners as many also contain chlorine.

Bromine

Bromine or bromide is the last of the halogen bullies and is extremely toxic. Bromide is found in pesticides and insecticides so it ends up on our food. It is also found in a variety of food products including some energy drinks, baked goods, bread and some medications.

Although potassium bromate (a bromine compound) was banned in the UK in 1990, it is still used in bakery products in the US. In 1999 the International Agency for Research on Cancer determined potassium bromate as a possible human carcinogen. Various studies have linked it to a myriad of health problems – from disrupting the genetic material in cells, to malignant tumours in the thyroid.

Other bromine compounds such as brominated vegetable oil (BVO) are used as emulsifiers in soft drinks – again recently banned in the UK but still on sale in the US. That said, a port authority surveillance exercise in 2014 revealed vast amounts of goods imported from the US still contained this bad halogen.

> ***Easy Step:*** Carefully read labels and avoid all products that contain bromide or brominated materials. Choose organic foods as much as possible to limit your exposure from bromide found in pesticides.

Bad Halogens are Everywhere

The biggest challenge with the bad halogens is that they are not just in our food or, for some of us, our water supply, they are added to the personal care products we use such as shampoo, conditioners, shower gels, soaps etc. and they are also in plastics, certain medications, fabrics, carpets, upholstery and mattresses.

Bad halogens have some useful properties such as disinfectants or fire retardants, which make them very appealing to a wide range of products and services, but this means that these bad halogens are then absorbed by the body from our everyday environment.

Ideally seek to minimise your exposure to these bad halogens wherever possible, read labels, and invest in a water filter. And increase your iodine intake, either from food or supplements (more on supplements in chapters 9 and 10). Iodine is a very powerful and positive element in the human body. So long as you have enough in your body it will help to top up what has been displaced by the bad halogen bullies.

Easy Step: Help your body out and give it more iodine – not only will this help your waistline by helping to stabilise your metabolism but it will also diminish the negative effects of the bad halogens as iodine helps to detoxify their harmful effects.

Mercury: The Deadly Toxins at the Dentist

Although not a bad halogen, mercury is another neurotoxin that we are constantly exposed to – often without us even knowing.

The British are internationally renowned for having bad teeth. In fact 84 per cent of British adults have one or more fillings and on average six missing teeth! And yet despite the stereotypes the US isn't much better; despite adding fluoride to the tap water, studies show the average American has seven missing teeth.

The challenge in the UK is that if you need a filling and visit your NHS dentist, unless you specify differently and pay a little extra, you will receive an amalgam filling. Amalgam fillings contain mercury which is seriously bad for our health. The United Nations has called for a ban on mercury and many countries, including Norway, Sweden, Denmark and Russia, have since banned the use of amalgam. In fact, the 2013 Minamata Convention on Mercury is a legally binding multilateral government agreement designed to protect human health and the environment from anthropogenic emissions and releases of mercury and mercury compounds. So why on earth are many dentists still putting this known carcinogen in our mouths?

The link between mercury fillings and mental health has been known for decades. In fact a Colorado State University study published in 1989 showed that dental amalgam fillings play a role in the cause of mental illness. The findings proved that 'comparisons between subjects with and without amalgam showed significant differences in subjective reports of mental health. Subjects who had amalgam fillings removed reported that symptoms of mental illness lessened or disappeared after removal.'

Mercury messes with our brains pure and simple. If you have amalgam fillings, every time you chew mercury vapours are released and research from the International Academy of Oral Medicine and Toxicology shows it can continue to be released up to 1.5 hours after eating. In fact, just one amalgam filling releases as much as 15 micrograms of mercury per day and, as most people have more than one filling, this soon adds up, slowly poisoning our bodies and our brains.

In fact, mercury causes havoc throughout our body and its impact extends far beyond mental health problems. It makes us fat too! It binds with iodine rendering it useless (similar to what the bad halogens do) and this causes low thyroid function which triggers weight gain. It causes mutations in our good gut flora, which is our first line of defence against disease, helping us to maintain a healthy weight and protecting our brains. Mercury also displaces magnesium – another crucial micronutrient for mental health. It binds with selenium, depleting us of this vital mineral, and interferes with the action of vitamin C and B12 causing a rise in homocysteine (a waste by-product produced when our cells metabolise protein). In short, mercury is linked to a whole host of health disorders from Alzheimer's, heart attacks, obesity, diabetes, cancer and many more. It has no place in the human body and we must do whatever we can to get rid of it.

If you live in the UK you can ask your dentist to remove your amalgam fillings but this is not routinely offered on the NHS. A funding request will be sent away to a dental panel who decide whether or not they will cover the cost of your treatment. On average, there is a 30 per cent success rate for funding requests so to boost your chances it may be an idea to ask your GP for a heavy metal toxin test. This will analyse your blood for traces of mercury and other heavy metals. If it comes back positive, that will provide support for your NHS treatment. Elevated calcium levels in your blood may also improve your chances.

For readers who do not have a state-funded health service or their GPs won't authorise the tests, then it might be an idea to save up the money to have your fillings replaced with a safer composite resin. And if you are totally strapped for cash, then chlorella supplements (more on that in chapter 9) is the next best thing. Chlorella is a proven heavy metal detoxing agent and it will help remove mercury and other toxins from your body. Algin is another good option – it is found in brown algae and both these algae help to absorb mercury in the colon, preventing it from being reabsorbed in the colon walls.

Easy Step: At the very least NEVER agree to another amalgam metal filling, always pay the small extra payment for the safer, white, non-metallic composite resin. Not only do they look better but they don't contain any mercury.

Mercury is also used as a preservative in many vaccines including the flu jab that many of us get every year. It's used in haemorrhoid creams, ear ointments – even contact lens solutions and nasal sprays. It is also in certain beauty creams. It is absolutely essential you ask your doctor or pharmacist for confirmation of the ingredients of any medicine or personal care product you buy as even tiny amounts of this heavy metal can damage our health.

Chapter 6: Macronutrients vs Micronutrients

'The food you eat can be either the safest and most powerful form of medicine or the slowest form of poison.'

– Ann Wigmore

According to the Food Standards Agency (FSA) in the UK this is what we need to 'eat well' (Figure 6.1). It is a graphic that illustrates what food groups we need to eat for health and in what proportion. At first glance this looks logical. It certainly ties in with what we have been repeatedly told by health experts for years.

Figure 6.1: What we should be eating as a proportion of our diet according to the FSA ('Eatwell Plate')

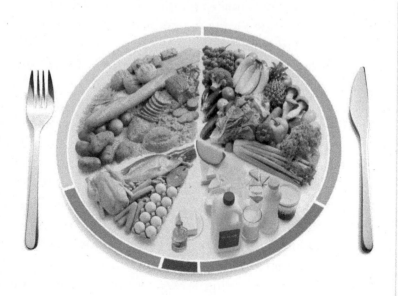

But there are a few problems with these food groups in Figure 6.1. First, there is no distinction made about the quality of these foods. Home-grown or organic fruit and vegetables are infinitely more nutritious than industrially grown, non-organic produce. Traditionally farmed, preferably organic meat is a world away in terms of nutritional content and purity to the factory-farmed alternative, wrapped in plastic and so often chosen by the time-strapped working woman.

This means that you may be eating what you believe to be the 'right' food and what our governments tell us is the 'right' food and still struggle with weight or mental health issues. And this delivers a double whammy because not only are you still fat, mad or both – but you are utterly bewildered and confused because nothing is changing despite your very best efforts.

Every overweight person on the planet believes they have 'tried everything'. We've all fibbed a little on that front but a study published in the *Obesity Research & Clinical Practice* journal found that it really is harder for today's adults to maintain the same weight as people 20 to 30 years ago, even at the same levels of food intake and exercise.

So any given person, in 2006, eating the same amount of calories, taking in the same quantities of macronutrients like protein and fat, and exercising the same amount as a person of the same age did in 1988, would have a body mass index (BMI) that was about 2.3 points higher. In other words, people today are about 10 per cent heavier than people were in the 1980s, even if they follow the exact same diet and exercise plans.

Which leads us to the second problem with the overemphasis on macronutrients – it fails to address the absolutely critical nature of micronutrients in our diet. Perhaps the assumption was that if we eat the right quantities of these macronutrients we would automatically have our micronutrient requirements taken care of. But that isn't happening because we don't appreciate the vast nutritional difference between foods in the various food groups depending on how they were grown or produced.

If the food we are eating lacks key micronutrients then

our body will lack the same key micronutrients. And it is this lack of micronutrients, together with an increase in exposure to various chemicals in food production and packaging, that is making it increasingly hard to lose weight. In addition, SSRI antidepressants are almost always linked to weight gain which makes it especially hard to lose weight if you are fat and mad!

Our food and medications are literally changing our physiology and our behaviour, making it harder and harder for us to stay sane and lose weight. So when your friend tells you that they really have tried everything, or when you really have tried everything – it's probably true! We need to eat the correct balance of minerals and vitamins for our brains and metabolism to function properly.

Our brain is never completely at rest; even when we are asleep the nervous system is still the most metabolically active organ in the body. This means our brain needs lots of energy and plenty of fuel in the form of nutrition. If we don't get that fuel our brain and metabolism don't function properly and yet we just put it down to lack of willpower or some other personal failing.

Stop! Stop beating yourself up and instead get yourself educated so you know about the macronutrients and the various food groups. And, perhaps more importantly, the specific micronutrients you need to ensure you get from the food you eat so you can lose weight and wean yourself off antidepressants.

Think of macronutrients as the petrol or diesel in your car. You need that fuel so you can get from A to B, but fuel is not enough to ensure you get where you are going safely. You need to make sure there is oil in the engine, enough brake fluid and that the electrics are all functioning properly. You need to make sure the wheels are aligned and balanced, and there is enough air in the tyres. These 'other' car maintenance issues are easily forgotten about and yet if you ignore them completely it won't matter how much petrol you have in the tank, your car will eventually break down. Your body is the same – it may not happen today, or tomorrow, but without micronutrients your body is going to break down. Without adequate micronutrients physical and mental illness is inevitable.

It is assumed that if we eat a varied diet made up of the elements on the 'Eatwell Plate' in Figure 6.1 above, then we will automatically get the micronutrients we need. The problem is that most of us don't eat the right proportions of these various food groups – eating too much processed meat, bread, pasta, starchy or sugary products because it's quick and easy. And even if we do follow these guidelines the nutritional value derived from these food groups varies considerably depending on where you buy your food and how it was produced. We may have access to more food and greater variety than our grandparents did, but often that food is less nutritious. And that is having a massive impact on our physical and mental well-being. Plus, to make matters worse, most food doesn't list micronutrient content on the label so it's not easy to figure out if we are getting the right amounts of what we need. Most food labels only specify the macronutrient content, i.e. how many calories are in the product, fat, carbohydrate, fibre, protein and salt. Some will use a traffic light system of red for bad/unhealthy, amber for average and green for good/healthy, but that doesn't help us to know if we are getting enough micronutrients.

Going back to the car analogy and taking it a little further, when the oil in your car gets dirty and clogged up, metal erosion caused by gas burn creates tiny corrosive particles that make the oil more acidic. This acidic oil damages the engine if it is not replaced with clean oil. Our brain is the exact same. Because our brain is rapidly metabolising nutrients it produces free radicals and lipid peroxidation, which means parts of the brain begin to oxidise or corrode resulting in cell damage. This oxidation is the leading cause of mental disorders and studies now show it is linked to Alzheimer's, Parkinson's and other diseases which destroy the structure of the brain – just like dirty oil damages a car's engine. Our brain needs a regular 'oil change' to replace the damaged cells. All components of the brain are constantly being replaced – some faster than others. Omega-3 fatty acids

(DHA) are replaced within just a couple of weeks. If we do not eat enough oily fish or take omega-3 supplements, our brain begins to change structure and starts to malfunction as one of its vital components is missing. Think about that for a moment – a deficiency of omega-3 fatty acids for just two weeks is enough to kick-start brain malfunction, and the first sign of this is usually exhibited in altered mood and a change in our behaviour.

Many studies over the years have linked diet with behaviour. But we know this ourselves – we don't need doctors in white coats telling us that what we eat changes behaviour. Anyone who has children or spent time with kids after a birthday party knows that after gorging themselves on pizza, processed burgers, sweeties and gallons of fizzy drinks they go nuts! It's almost like we have to peel them off the ceiling and their hyperactivity can last several exhausting hours!

And we've known the connection for a very long time despite what some experts have been telling us. Way back in 1910 Dr George M. Gould wrote in one of his study papers,

For several years it has been growing clearer to me that many patients do not get well because they live too exclusively on sugary and starchy foods...I have asked the parents of such children to stop them in their use of all sweets, and most starches, and almost immediately there was a most gratifying disappearance of the 'nervousness,' fickleness of appetite, colds, and vague manifold ailments.

Over 100 years ago this medical doctor made the connection between certain foods and child hyperactivity. Today that observation is increasingly swept away in favour of a drug that can be sold indefinitely. Diagnosis of ADHD soared by 43 per cent in the US during the first decade of this century. Today more than one in ten young people are diagnosed with ADHD and prescribed a pill when actually a change of diet would probably deliver far superior results.

Other studies showed that hyperglycaemia (too much

glucose in the blood) can cause symptoms such as anxiety, hysteria and even psychosis. In fact, diet has now been linked with violence and nutrient-poor Western diets contribute to psychopathology. A study published in the *Oxford Journal of Nutrition* in 2002, looking at the influence of supplements on antisocial behaviour in young adult prisoners, showed a 35 per cent reduction in violent acts when prisoners were given a daily multivitamin as well as omega-3 fatty acids. Another Dutch study showed that aggressive behaviour in prisoners was linked to deficiencies in omega-3 and that low levels of magnesium and zinc are also associated with hyperactive behaviour, impaired brain development and cognitive dysfunction.

Epidemiological researchers (scientists who study patterns, causes and effects of health and disease) have published many studies over the years which show how changes in our diet (especially in the Western world over the last century) have resulted in significantly lower micronutrient intake than our ancestors.

We are simply not consuming enough vitamins and minerals any more, which makes it harder for us to lose weight. It's also affecting our behaviour – making many of us mad!

In the remainder of this chapter we will explore diet in more detail – looking at each macronutrient or food group in turn. The purpose is to get clearer about each one, what's in each one that is essential for health, and how to ensure we get the best possible quality. I'll also reiterate what's actually happening in each group in terms of production so we have a better understanding of exactly what we are eating. The five macronutrient food groups we will cover are:

- Fruit and vegetables
- Protein (meat, fish and eggs)
- Carbohydrate (bread, rice, potatoes, pasta, cereal and sugars)
- Dairy
- Fats and oils

Fruit and Vegetables

Fruit and vegetables are an important source of minerals and vitamins and a rich source of antioxidants, which help protect the body from oxidative damage. They contain thousands of biologically active phytochemicals that interact in a number of ways to prevent disease and promote health. The best way to take advantage of these complex interactions is to eat a variety of fruit and vegetables every day.

Antioxidants (the main ones being vitamins A, C and E) in fruit and vegetables are incredibly important for human health because antioxidants 'clean' our cells and tissues. When our cells get inflamed (due to stress or toxins) fluid spills out of blood vessels and into the space between cells, creating a build-up of what are called 'free radicals'. You've probably heard free radicals mentioned on TV adverts promoting anti-ageing products – they are uncharged molecules which cause oxidation or cell breakdown. These wee bandits steal electrons from other cells, leaving them damaged and vulnerable to ageing and disease. Antioxidants soak up free radicals like a dry sponge soaking up dirty water. They are white knights that rescue us from the ongoing damage caused by these pesky free radicals.

But finding a few extra wrinkles is the least of our worries. In 2015 scientists at the Centre for Addiction and Mental Health in Toronto published research findings demonstrating that excessive inflammation in brain cells interferes with the way neurons communicate with each other. Brain scans confirmed that depressed patients showed over a third more brain cell inflammation than patients with no mental illness. But the Canadians are not alone in linking depression to cellular inflammation and you can find the sources for a whole bunch of peer-reviewed research papers at the back of the book if you fancy a spot of light bedtime reading!

Scientists and medics agree that most illness starts with inflammation. Pain, obesity, ADHD, diabetes, heart disease, stroke, migraines, thyroid issues, dental issues, cancer and depression all start with an inflammatory reaction. Fruits and vegetables rich in antioxidants are therefore essential for minimising inflammation and helping the body heal itself by removing highly damaging free radicals.

In the UK we are encouraged to eat '5 a day'. In other words, we are encouraged to eat at least five portions of fruit or vegetables every day, but the quality of those five a day *really* does matter. Also, potatoes don't count in your five a day. The whole fruit or vegetable is always preferable to processed or juiced. But even then you may not be eating what you think you are eating...

The ugly truth behind 'fresh' fruit and vegetables

The first time I noticed just how much fruit and vegetable production had changed, certainly from my early days running down to the greengrocer for my granny, was when I was visiting supermarkets on Vancouver Island in 2005. I was working on a marketing project with a leading Canadian retailer and had the privilege of being ushered around their stores to see the way food was promoted on the Pacific Coast. I still remember seeing the apples on display at the front of the store – they were magnificent. Each perfect fruit was cartoon red – straight out of a scene from *Snow White and the Seven Dwarfs*. Glistening under the carefully designed overhead lighting and displayed with military precision, these apples were so polished I initially thought they were fake – a marketing display only. To check, I picked one up to see if they were real.

I was quite taken aback and turned to the manager who was looking a little confused. 'Wow, these look amazing – are they locally produced?' I thought they must have been imported given it was February with sub-zero temperatures outside. He replied, 'Yes. We have a great produce team who look after our fruit storage.' I wondered what on earth he meant. Did they tuck them up in bed at night and sing lullabies to the apples, or were they individually polished every evening by the hands of virgins? Turns out the apples were sprayed every night but apparently the real magic occurred long before the fruit arrived in the store.

In North America, apples generally ripen between August and September. They are picked when slightly unripe, sprayed with a chemical called 1-methylcyclopropene (1-MCP), waxed (with a petroleum-based agent), boxed, stacked on pallets and then kept in a cold store for up to 12 months! The spray is known as 'SmartFresh' and in 2011 the Canadian government expanded this treatment so that apples can now be sprayed with this chemical up to four times during storage.

So when you select your delicious-looking apples from your supermarket, thinking you are 'doing the right thing' and eating healthily, you are possibly buying an apple that was picked over a year ago! SmartFresh is now used on a wide range of fruits and vegetables in over 26 countries, including the UK, US and Australia. So the fresh produce you are buying in the local supermarket is actually not that 'fresh' at all.

Fruit and vegetables contain the maximum nutritional value the moment they are harvested. The longer they are in storage the more their nutritional value deteriorates. Studies show SmartFresh reduces the antioxidant (vitamin) levels in fruits. Petroleum-based wax, used to preserve fruit and vegetables, is also used on other produce including cucumbers, potatoes, oranges, bell peppers, limes, lemons, aubergines and courgettes. This coating locks in any pesticides and herbicides used when growing the plants, making it very difficult to remove when washing at home. Even if you peel your fruit or vegetables they have often been sitting in storage so long that the pesticides have soaked all the way through, so even if you remove the skin you are probably still eating pesticide residue.

This is very different from the odd-shaped, dirt-caked fruit and vegetables my granny bought in brown paper bags from the local greengrocer. There were no preservatives so we only ate what was in season. No one worried about the 'air miles' the food travelled because it didn't travel far. It couldn't travel far because there were no preservatives to keep it in tip-top condition. We knew what we were eating was fresh because otherwise it would be rotten within days. The fruits and vegetables my granny ate delivered the micronutrients she needed but the mass-produced, mass-preserved, sprayed and polished 'fresh' produce available in many supermarkets may not.

A landmark study published in 2004 in *The American College of Nutrition* journal showed a 'reliable decline' in the amount of protein, calcium, phosphorus, iron, vitamin B2 and vitamin C found in fruit and vegetables over the past 50 years. Comparing the nutritional data of produce from 1950 to the nutritional data of produce in 1999, scientists reported declines in other nutrients such as magnesium, zinc, vitamin B6 and vitamin E.

The Organic Consumers Association in the US cites several other studies with similar findings: a Kushi Institute analysis of nutrient data from 1975 to 1997 found that the average calcium levels in 12 fresh vegetables dropped 27 per cent; iron levels dropped 37 per cent; vitamin A levels dropped 21 per cent; and vitamin C levels dropped 30 per cent. A similar study of British nutrient data from 1930 to 1980, published in the *British Food Journal*, found that in 20 vegetables the average calcium content had declined 19 per cent; iron had dropped by 22 per cent; and potassium by 14 per cent. Yet another study concluded that we would have to eat eight oranges today to get the same amount of vitamin C our grandparents received from just one orange.

And to make matters worse it's not just the drop in micronutrients. Many of the pre-packed produce we have come to rely on, such as mixed salad leaves, are washed in chlorine (one of the bad halogens) before being packed in modified atmospheric packaging. This method of preparation and packaging also reduces the amount of oxygen in the bag while filling it with carbon dioxide. Research from the Rome Institute of Food and Nutrition shows that salad preserved using this method loses its antioxidants just as quickly as lettuce left to go off naturally. In other words, by the time the leaves are eaten they may still look 'fresh' but their micronutrient value is almost non-existent.

Don't get me wrong, it would be ludicrous to suggest that all fruit and vegetables today have very little nutrition, and we would be crazy to stop eating them. But the hard facts speak for themselves. The fresh produce enjoyed by our grandparents was substantially more nutritious than the fresh produce we eat today.

So, where possible:

1. Grow your own.

If that's not possible, or you don't have the time or inclination, then…

2. Source a local producer that grows fruit and vegetables traditionally and buy direct. Many farm shops now offer online ordering and delivery options; check out the 'pick your own' venues – make a day of it and gather up some fresh 'in season' goodies. Farmers' markets are also a great place to buy locally produced fresh fruit and vegetables.

If that's not possible or you don't have the time, then…

3. Buy organic.

Often organic produce is more expensive so you may have to buy a little less. If there are limited organic options in your area, then…

4. Take dietary supplements to ensure you are getting the necessary micronutrients.

Protein

The word 'protein' comes from the Greek word for 'first' (*protos*), indicating its role as the building block of life. It is part of every cell in our body. Aside from water, protein is the most abundant compound found in the human body. No other macronutrient plays as many different roles in keeping us alive and healthy. It is essential for growth and repair in everything from our muscles to our bones, skin, tendons, hair, eyes and more. Without protein we would lack the enzymes and hormones we need for metabolism, digestion and other important processes.

The main sources of protein are meat, fish and eggs. But again, the nutritional value depends on the quality of the protein you eat.

Meat

We've already discussed many of the problems with industrial farming when it comes to meat production. Let's take a closer look at chicken – fast becoming the meat of choice for many Western families. Again we have been told by health experts and government officials to cut down our red meat consumption and switch to white meat, such as chicken, instead. As a result, British consumers eat an average of 31kg of chicken per person per year – more than any other European country. Even the beef-loving Americans have switched their meat preference, and since 2014 Americans are now eating more chicken than beef.

So what's the problem? White meat is supposed to be lower in fat but cheap chicken is often not. Chickens bred for meat are arguably the most genetically manipulated of all animals, forced to grow 65 times faster than their bodies normally would. As mentioned in chapter 1, this means that the fat content in chicken has increased from 2 per cent to 22 per cent in just 30 years. Intensively reared chickens (and pigs) are also often fed genetically modified soy and corn which is very high in omega-6 and this has also altered the balance of vital fatty acids in chicken and pork, which means you are almost certainly eating too much omega-6 and not enough omega-3. Remember we should be consuming 1:3 omega-3 to omega-6 but we are actually consuming 1:16, leading to inflammation and mental dysfunction. And without good-quality fruit and vegetables full of antioxidants to fight those free radicals, inflammation can have serious knock-on effects on our health.

In every Western nation chickens are produced in much the same way. If you would like to see the process then Google 'Animal Equality: The unbelievable life of baby chicks', although I warn you – you may never eat cheap chicken again! Batches of eggs arranged in rows ride along a conveyor belt. A machine then punctures each egg and injects a mixture of vaccines and antibiotics into the unborn chick inside the egg. As we've already discussed, this blanket use of antibiotics is causing a serious problem because it is creating superbugs that are no longer responding to antibiotics.

These vaccines contain genetically modified serotypes (microorganisms) and bacteria and are part of a veterinary vaccine market valued at $5.6 billion (2015) and forecast to rise to over $7 billion by 2020. Although legally limited in the UK and parts of Europe, blanket use of antibiotics is still rife in the US, Asia and China.

Once injected with the chemical cocktail the chicks will hatch three days later. They are often reared in gigantic overcrowded sheds, packed in by the thousands with no room to move, often sitting on filthy, manure-laden floors. 'Free range' is often completely meaningless in food marketing since almost all chickens reared for meat are uncaged. It's a marketing ploy to reassure us that the chicken on our plate had a happy (albeit short) life before it was the Sunday roast. If you buy cheap chicken – it's pretty safe to assume it didn't have a happy life. Nutritionally this fast, mass-produced chicken provides nowhere near the nutritional value of genuinely free-range, corn-fed and organic chicken.

And do we really know where our chicken comes from? The price of chicken produced in different geographical markets can vary. When I was in a senior role at a large UK food processors it was common practice to substitute British chicken with foreign chicken. For example, Brazilian chicken is almost half as expensive as Scottish-raised poultry because they often don't have higher welfare standards or the same regulation. So when the big retailers forced a two for one promotion or supply of local chicken was low, the sales director and operations director would have one of their 'after-hours chats' to ensure the order was fulfilled even if the meat inside the packaging didn't match the origin information advertised on the label.

Unfortunately, this type of behaviour is not rare. Traceability of food is still relatively poor for those retailers who want it to be.

But it's often not just what's in chicken that causes the problems. Although banned in the EU, in the US chicken is also washed in chlorine (that bad halogen again). So, in the US, not only is the chicken meat chock-full of hormones, growth promoters and antibiotics, it's washed in a neurotoxin. Yummy!

Like all macronutrients the quality of the protein we eat matters. So, where possible:

1. Source a local, traditional meat producer who is using the old traditional rearing techniques and buy direct.

You may be able to find a local producer at a local farmers' market. Beef from cattle which eat grass (labelled as 'grass fed') is higher in conjugated linoleic acid (CLA) which has been linked to reducing fat in the body and therefore helps weight loss. Studies have indicated CLA also has potent cancer-fighting properties across a wide variety of tumours. It also lowers LDL (bad) cholesterol levels, prevents bone loss, hardening of the arteries and actually protects the brain. Beef *not* fed on grass can also be high in omega-6 which further amplifies the already significant omega-3: omega-6 imbalance. Unfortunately for US readers, in early 2016 the USDA revoked 'grass fed' meat labelling despite widespread support from farmers and consumers. This move, no doubt facilitated by powerful lobby groups keen to keep US consumers in the dark about the quality of meat they are eating, means that it will be next to impossible for US consumers to know if they are buying good-quality grass-fed beef with high animal welfare standards or mass-produced beef pumped full of growth hormones, antibiotics and steroids where animal welfare simply doesn't enter the equation.

Also consider switching to turkey. Most of us only consider eating turkey on Thanksgiving or at Christmas but it is packed full of tryptophan – an amino acid that helps produce serotonin (the happy hormone). Tryptophan also helps you sleep. Sleep deprivation is heavily linked to depression and weight problems – not least because we then binge on carbohydrates because we are so tired. Try eating turkey for dinner instead of chicken or beef. Make a turkey stir-fry and add some cashew nuts – also high in tryptophan. Turkey is lower in fat and is often cheaper than buying chicken breasts in the supermarkets. Consider buying a whole one, carve it into pieces and freeze it. The carcase can also be used to make a great stock for soups and sauces. If you still prefer chicken then go for the dark chicken meat – it's higher in nutrients than white breast meat – and also less expensive. Myoglobin (an oxygen-carrying protein) gives dark meat its colour and is richer in zinc, iron, vitamins: A, K, B6, B12, niacin, folic acid, pantothenic acid and minerals like selenium and phosphorus. Again – all essential micronutrients for brain health.

It's not for everyone but consider putting offal such as liver back on the menu. Liver is incredibly high in B vitamins (B12, folic acid, niacin) and selenium, choline and iron – the big brain-boosting vitamins which help to maintain our mental well-being. Plus it's incredibly cheap because it's fallen out of fashion.

If sourcing a local traditional meat producer is not possible or you don't want to invest the time, then...

2. Buy organic.

Again you may need to buy a little less but there will be none of the chemical residues found in mass-produced meat.

If there are limited organic options in your area, then at least...

3. Reduce, and in some cases eliminate, the amount of processed meat you eat.

In 2015 the World Health Organization (WHO) announced that processed meats cause cancer. However, not all processed meats are created equal. The problem with Western processed meats are the nitrates used as preservatives, which are used to speed up the curing process and add colour. Traditional cured meats are not produced in this way – and that might explain why cancer statistics in Italy and Spain are far lower than, say, the UK and US. Traditional prosciutto-style meat produced in the Mediterranean region (such as Parma ham) is dried and aged for at least 18 months using only salt as a curing agent. Plus the pigs are traditionally raised on a native diet. Similarly, pancetta is salt cured and preserved using herbs and spices. Another factor missing from the WHO report is the omega-3 to omega-6 ratio in the Western diet which is compounding this problem. The Spanish and Italians eat far more omega-3-rich foods (oils and fish) than those in the UK or US – so any nitrates that are present in their diet from eating processed meat are more easily mitigated by the anti-inflammatory effect of the high omega-3 fatty acids they consume.

If you are going to buy processed meat such as bacon and sausages, buy it from your local butcher and cut out the highly processed meats such as hot dogs or dodgy beefburgers. Red 2G (listed in the ingredients as E128) is red dye extracted from coal tar. It is often added to burgers and sausages and it converts to aniline, which is a carcinogen, once inside the body.

My advice is simple. If you do eat meat – buy quality, traditionally produced or organic products. If you have to buy a little less, then buy a little less and simply add more vegetables to your plate – job done!

Fish

Fish is also a great source of protein but its other nutritional qualities are what really set it apart. Unfortunately, we eat two-thirds less fish than we did 50 years ago.

In my granny's day fish was a regular part of the Scottish diet. It was cheap and easily available. In fact, you could buy it straight from the fishing boats on the Clyde in the days when the Clyde was teeming with herring, plaice, cod, sole and other tasty varieties. She would regularly use whatever she could get locally to make her delicious Cullen skink (Scottish fish chowder), fish pie or we had our Saturday night favourite – fish and chips from the chippie straight out of the newspaper with plenty of salt and vinegar.

Like so many places around the world, the introduction of trawling on the Clyde radically altered the river ecosystem. Prawn and scallop dredging meant that the larger, older fish disappeared, which further devastated local fish stocks. Needless to say, the price of fish soon began to rise.

Plus tastes began to change. The weekend treat of fish and chips soon gave way to Quarter-Pounders, Whoppers and buckets of chicken as American fast-food outlets like McDonald's, Burger King and KFC expanded outside the US. All washed down with a tsunami of fizzy drink or sugar-laden milkshake.

The nutritional value of the locally sourced fish and chips, bread and butter and a nice cup of tea that my granny enjoyed while watching *The Generation Game* on a Saturday night to the fast-food junk we consume today is like comparing night and day.

Ironically, the population of some of the major fish-producing countries don't eat enough fish. Scotland, for example, is a major producer of farmed salmon, second only to Norway and Canada. And yet Scots still don't eat anywhere near enough fish. Just 27 per cent of Scottish women eat one portion of oily fish, rich in omega-3, per week. Forty per cent of Canadians also don't get enough of this essential fatty acid.

However, Norwegians do eat fish – lots of fish – and that probably helps to explain why mental illness is far lower in Norway than other European countries, Canada and the US. In fact, a Norwegian study conducted by researchers at the University of Oslo showed that eating just 10g of fish per day makes your mind sharper. A later Dutch study demonstrated that it was the elevated omega-3 levels in the blood from eating fish that made study participants respond quicker to mental skills tests. Granny always said fish is brain food – and again it looks like she was right.

As with meat, the quality of your fish matters so, where possible:

1. Source a local sustainable supplier so you know where your fish is coming from.

Food fraud is a major issue with fish. In fact, a recent study published by Oceana in the US showed that 44 per cent of retail outlets in the US sold mislabelled fish. This means cheaper species sold in place of more expensive ones. It can also mean trawler-caught fish sold as line-caught fish, farmed sold as 'wild' or sustainably sourced when it really isn't. Adulteration is also rife. Pink colouring is used to make farmed fish look like wild fish. And the new kid on the block is genetically modified salmon – which has just been approved by the FDA in the US. This is salmon with a growth hormone gene added – so it grows to a gigantic size compared to regular salmon. This fish does not need to be labelled as GM so consumers won't know they are eating genetically modified fish.

Ideally buy your fish from someone you know and trust who can help to ensure you get the best-quality, sustainable fish you can.

If that's not possible, or you don't have the time or inclination to find a reputable fish supplier...

2. Read the labelling carefully and only buy fish that is sustainably caught.

Of course, fraudulent mislabelling and changes to labelling laws such as the changes to grass-fed beef labelling in the US will make this harder and harder.

If there are limited sustainably sourced fish options available to you, then...

3. Take dietary supplements to ensure you are getting the necessary micronutrients.

Despite having to run the gauntlet when buying fish these days – eating fish is still by far the best way to ensure we are getting a steady amount of omega-3. The omega-3 in fish (EPA and DHA) is different from the ALA in plant-derived omega-3, which makes fish an absolutely critical element in our diet. Even for vegetarians! Increasing intake of omega-3 (and/or decreasing intake of omega-6) is a recommended and proven treatment for a wide variety of conditions from heightened aggression, anxiety, allergies, bipolar disorder, weight issues, heart disease and depression.

I simply can't stress enough the importance of eating fish so that you get the right amount of omega-3 in your diet.

Eggs

Back in the 1960s we were told to 'Go to work on an egg' as our government promoted eggs as the preferred breakfast of champions. Of course, this was long before the cereal giants gained a starring role in our corner shops, grocery stores and supermarket aisles. Expensive TV advertising campaigns, together with the indoctrination of the 'fat is bad' message promoted by health authorities in the 1980s, encouraged us to swap our egg and soldiers for Corn Flakes, Rice Krispies or other more sugary breakfast cereal varieties.

The thing is researchers from Cambridge University have since discovered that going to work on an egg is still by far the best advice. They looked at how nutrients in eggs affect the brain cells that keep us awake and burn calories. Their research, published in the journal *Neuron*, showed that eating eggs triggered the release of orexin, a neuropeptide that regulates wakefulness and appetite. So eating eggs helps to keep us awake and burn more calories, sharpen the mind and makes us feel less tired and lethargic. Interestingly, the researchers also found that eating breakfast cereals and sugar had the opposite effect – as these blocked the release of orexin.

Eggs have had such a bad press over the years – mainly due to government advice on cholesterol. But as we explored in chapter 2, the change to cholesterol advice in 2004 turned out to benefit no one other than the drug companies who could sell more products. Other health scares such as the one created by UK MP Edwina Currie haven't helped the egg's reputation. In the early 1980s Currie said that, 'Most of the egg production in this country, sadly, is now affected with salmonella'. Her poorly educated statement led to a 60 per cent crash in the demand for eggs.

Yet despite it all, research conclusively demonstrates that eggs are good for our physical and mental health. Many nutritionists now consider eggs a 'superfood' as they are one of the most nutrient-dense foods. A study published in the journal *Nutrition and Food Science* in 2010 analysed 71 research papers that examined the nutritional composition of eggs and their role in the diet. They found that eggs are not only low in calories (just 80 calories per average egg) but packed full of antioxidants and vital nutrients such as selenium, vitamin B12, vitamin D and choline.

Choline is a powerhouse nutrient that you've probably never even heard of. In 1998 the Institute of Medicine recognised choline as an essential micronutrient. It supports the formation of S-adenosylmethionine (SAM-e) which helps neurotransmitters function properly in the brain. Put simply – we need choline for proper mental function and eggs are one of the best sources. Choline works by stimulating the production of the neurotransmitter 'acetylcholine' which is responsible for memory, mental clarity and connections between neurons. Unfortunately studies show that 90 per cent of people are not getting an adequate intake in their diet – probably because they've turned their back on the humble little egg.

Just one egg also provides 20 per cent of the recommended daily allowance of vitamin D – another nutrient vital for our health. In fact, all the nutrients found in a single egg are absolutely vital for mental health and weight loss.

As with all the food groups we've discussed so far, the quality of your eggs matters so, where possible:

1. Produce your own.

If you have a garden or live in a rural area then it's very easy to keep chickens and produce your own eggs. You will need a little 'hen house' to keep them safe from predators at night but simply let them out through the day. It's relaxing just watching them scratch about in the garden and equally rewarding to eat your very own eggs. Plus you can sell the excess to your neighbours or donate to a local food bank.

If that's not possible, or you don't have the time or inclination to rear your own chickens…

2. Find someone else who does. Buy locally from an organic, free-range producer.

For example, I live on the outskirts of Glasgow – the biggest city in Scotland – and I can still buy my eggs locally. I buy mine from the local post office! They are actually produced by a farmer just down the road from where I live. I often see his hens happily scratching around his yard as I drive past. They are free to roam around and eat grubs and bugs that they find in the yard. The yolks in these eggs are a rich, vibrant yellow and they taste delicious. And, they are often cheaper than buying them in the shops and I like the fact that I'm helping to support one of my neighbours. It's a win-win!

If that's not possible, or you don't have the time or inclination to find a local organic egg producer…

3. Buy organic, free-range eggs (never caged eggs).

Supermarket eggs, even organic or free range, are often weeks old even though they are marketed as fresh. You can always tell how fresh an egg is by how watery the whites are. Fresh eggs have stiff, gloopy whites and freshly laid eggs straight from the farm are slightly opaque in colour. However, if you can't get those then organic, free-range eggs are the next best thing.

Following the salmonella furore in the UK, vaccination for salmonella was introduced in 1998. This vaccination was backed by the new British Lion mark. Every egg with this mark – even organic eggs – means the hen that laid it has been vaccinated against salmonella. But the vaccination is not needed when the birds are raised in a genuine free-range environment and fed a natural diet.

If there are limited free-range, organic options or you just don't like eggs, then…

4. Take dietary supplements to ensure you are getting the necessary micronutrients.

Carbohydrate

Carbohydrates are the body's main source of energy. They are easily digested and broken down into glucose, which the body then uses to perform numerous functions. Carbohydrates are separated into simple carbohydrates (sugar), complex carbohydrates (fibre) and starch. Carbohydrates are needed for the central nervous system, the kidneys, the brain and the muscles (including the heart) to function properly.

The main sources of carbohydrate are bread, rice, potatoes, pasta, cereals and sugar. I'll cover a few of the key issues with some of these foods below.

Bread (and bakery goods)

We eat a lot of bread. In the UK we buy around 12 million loaves of bread a day – 76 per cent of which is white. It should contain flour, water and a dash of yeast but commercial breads often contain much more.

Once again, the nutritional value of bread will depend on the quality of the ingredients that make that bread. All bread is not equal. The mass-produced bread we grab from the supermarket 'in-house' bakery because we think it's wholesome and fresh is often not and it's significantly less nutritious than the bread my granny used to knock up in her kitchen on a Sunday afternoon.

Following the Second World War, plant breeders developed hybrid strains of wheat that responded positively to chemical fertilisers, herbicides and pesticides to deliver higher yields. The push to greater quantity and higher protein content came at the expense of vital minerals and vitamins usually found in the grain. These hybrid wheat varieties now have 30 to 40 per cent less iron, zinc and magnesium than strains grown 40 years ago. When bread is less nutritious we eat more, which is undoubtedly fuelling the fat part of the mad fat epidemic.

Chemical fertilisers containing sulphur and nitrogen added to boost yield late in the growing cycle means that the resulting flour has nearly double the wheat protein, known as omega-gliadins. Unlike the wonderful omega-3, omega-gliadins can trigger certain inflammatory reactions in the gut. Remember inflammation is a precursor to a whole range of serious illnesses, so anything that causes inflammation is bad! It's no surprise that more and more people are finding that bread doesn't agree with them. But once again, it's all about quality. Often it is the chemicals, additives and the way the bread is made that is making people feel bloated and sick.

The bread-making process is very different from the way my granny made a loaf. In the 1960s the Chorleywood bread process was invented and it is still the way most bread is made to this day. Its attraction to commercial bread making was simple – speed.

High speed mixing, a plethora of additives and increased yeast have done away with fermentation time. Before Chorleywood a baker would mix the dough and then leave it for a while to let the dough rise (or ferment). Most bread was therefore made in two stages over 12–16 hours. Time improved the dough, making it easier to handle and taste better. Plus the time to ferment neutralises that problematic wheat protein that can trigger inflammation and trigger bowel disease and other autoimmune and inflammatory reactions to gluten.

Chorleywood may have been a triumph for efficiency and profitability but it was not a triumph for bread quality, flavour or our health. Today, most bread is made from 'no time dough' – moving from raw flour to wrapped loaf in under three hours.

And to add insult to injury some bakers are now adding more and more substances to ensure your loaf maintains its pretence of being fresh for that little bit longer! These additives include potassium bromate (that bad halogen again), azodicarbonamide, L-cysteine hydrochloride, sodium stearoyl-2-lactylate and so on – the list is long. For the time being, the first two in that list are banned in the UK, but for how long? Bread manufacturers are allowed to group all the nasty additives under bland headings such as 'flour treatment agent', 'emulsifier' or 'improvers'.

So not only is modern commercial bread less nutritious than it could be, it is laced with undeclared additions and fermented for so little time that it clogs up our guts. Hardly the winning food group we have been assured it is.

Often, like many things in life, it comes down to money. There are huge margins to be made from products that require flour, water and little else! Bakery items too have huge financial potential because the raw ingredients are so cheap and the finished product can be sold for considerably more.

I still remember sitting in a bar on Île Saint-Louis with my best friend, sipping Sancerre and putting the world to rights on a well-earned girlie weekend to Paris. I received a call from my

CEO asking me to make a factory closure announcement on the Monday and that there may be 'some press fallout' to deal with. Our parent company (the largest sugar-producing company in the world) had decided to relocate UK bakery operations to Romania due to the low-cost benefits of producing our cakes and desserts in Eastern Europe. People were willing to work for a fraction of what British workers were paid and there was no threat of unionisation.

I couldn't believe what I was hearing. I had visited Romania on a few reconnaissance trips under the impression that we were expanding our operations – not planning to shut down factories in the UK. Romania was emerging from very difficult political times and it was a dangerous country back then, so I had to be escorted everywhere by a bodyguard. It was plain to see why big food companies wanted to set up shop there – cheap land, hardly any taxes to pay, and a workforce that would work for peanuts. I was excited about the plans because it would give Romanian people work and help to develop the country further. Little did I know that the board had other plans – they were not expanding! Instead they were relocating all operations to Romania so they could increase profit with zero thought for the communities they were going to leave high and dry in the UK. Our factory was based in a working-class community, a region that was already struggling with mass unemployment. A thousand people depended on our plant. Most lived in the local town and were often the sole breadwinner, so the ramifications of factory closure would extend far beyond the workforce. The closure would affect everyone, including the local shops and businesses where employees would spend their wages.

I don't know if it was because I was taken by surprise, blind rage or maybe the Sancerre kicking in, but in true Glasgow-style I told my boss to 'F**k off' and hung up. I took a huge gulp of wine, turned to my friend and said, 'I've just been sacked.' As the minutes passed the consequences of my actions started to sink in. As a single parent with a mortgage and the same debt everyone else had I realised it wasn't the smartest move in my career and that I was probably facing some tough times ahead, but I was so angry. I felt totally betrayed – I had reassured so many people in the factory that it was just an expansion, they trusted me and I trusted the board when they told *me* it was an expansion. There was no way I could stand up and tell the workers that it had all been a lie. So, I accepted my fate, polished off the bottle of wine we had and ordered another. Apparently I was singing alongside the pianist in Le Boeuf sur le Toit, a cosy art deco jazz restaurant just off Champs-Élysées later that evening – although I have to admit I don't remember!

As these things often do – it all worked out for the best. I had been growing uneasy about the company for some time. They manufactured a wide range of cake and dessert products for British and European supermarkets. We also held the licence to manufacture low-fat cake products for the biggest diet food brand in the world – a global giant with $1.7 billion turnover each year. These products sold very well and were listed in all the major supermarkets. Millions of British women were members of their slimming club so they trusted the brand and therefore trusted the products sold under their logo.

The main criterion for food sold under this brand was 'low fat'. Focus group studies showed that only 20 per cent of women read the back of the packaging so it didn't really matter about the other ingredients. All most consumers cared about was the blue 'low-fat' branding – written in big bold text on the front of the bakery item alongside the trusted logo.

When our new product development (NPD) team were challenged to create a new carrot cake recipe they came up against a whole range of issues because they needed to reduce the fat content in the cakes. The only way to get the cakes to look good and taste good, and withstand the long shelf life demanded by retailers, was to devise a cocktail of ingredients that would never appear in a carrot cake made by Delia Smith or Julia Child. The team worked really hard to keep the ingredients to a minimum and to stay as true to a real carrot cake as possible. But it was an impossible challenge. After a few focus group tasting sessions and screening by the brand owners, below is the final list of ingredients used to make the carrot cake – excluding the processing agents which do not need to be listed on the label:

Sugar, Fortified Wheat Flour [Wheat Flour, Calcium Carbonate, Iron, Niacin, Thiamine], Carrot (10%), Water, Humectánt: Glycerine, Pineapple, Shea Oil, Coconut, Raising Agents: Diphosphates, Potassium Bicarbonate, Citrus Fibre, Dried Egg Yolk, Dried Egg White, Glucose Syrup, Skimmed Milk Powder, Caramelised Sugar Syrup, Rapeseed Oil, Preservative: Potassium Sorbate, Gelling Agent: Pectin, Cinnamon, Tapioca Starch, Nutmeg, Dextrose, Fructose, Emulsifier: Sucrose Esters of Fatty Acids.

Notice that the first and therefore the largest quantity of ingredient is sugar. All 'low-fat' products are only 'low fat' because they are 'high sugar'. And no one loses weight eating bucketloads of sugar!

Look – I'm going to tell you a secret. YOU CAN'T LOSE WEIGHT EATING CAKE! Low fat or otherwise! It's a lie.

Carbohydrates are no different to any other food group – it's all about quality not quantity, so where possible:

1. Make your own.

It's dead easy to make bread. You don't even need a fancy bread maker. All you need is good-quality flour, some water, a dash of yeast and some time.

If you enjoy a little bit of cake every now and again – then again make it, using a genuinely low-fat, low-sugar recipe and organic ingredients.

If that's not possible, or you don't have the time or inclination to make your own bread or bakery items...

2. Find someone else who does. Buy locally from a small traditional bakery – ideally one that uses organic ingredients and old techniques.

If that's not possible, or you don't have a local producer…

3. Buy organic, wholegrain bread (not mass-market white) and cut back on the cakes. Honestly, if you're going to have cake, go for it and have a really nice piece of cake instead of those chemical-laden fake cakes that pretend to be healthy!

Cereal

Cereal has become the breakfast of choice for millions, not because it is good for us but because cereal giants have spent billions telling us how nutritious and convenient it is. Add the odd health scare or expert advice steering us away from our traditional breakfast foods and cereal producers have made a fortune.

A box of breakfast cereal can be produced with just 10 pence worth of grain. It is then sold for £2.50 or more per box! That's an extraordinary profit margin and certainly more exciting for food companies than the single-digit profits in meat and vegetables. It's easy to understand why big brands offer so many free toys and giveaways with boxes of cereals – the profits are gargantuan!

The 1980s was a great decade for cereal producers. Health scares such as salmonella turned us away from nutritious and cheap eggs. At much the same time we were told that fat was bad for us and UK and US governments advised us to eat more carbohydrates (including sugars). This advice was based on bogus clinical trial data. The study participants were made up of high-risk individuals or people with existing diseases so the results were immediately compromised. Oh, and have a guess who funded that research? Yep – you guessed it … pharmaceutical companies. Thirty-two years after these NHS guidelines were launched, Britain, the US and much of Western Europe is facing a mad fat epidemic of unprecedented proportions – with millions of patients requiring medication for mental health, obesity and diabetes. Great news for big pharma – terrible news for us.

It's a con – ditch the breakfast cereal altogether. Have an egg, porridge or home-made, wholegrain toast instead.

By now you should be getting the message – we need to be much more focused on what's in our food and the quality of our food, not just on how much fat or sugar we are eating, or how many portions of fruit and vegetables we are having each day. Quality really matters and it doesn't have to cost more to get. We need to eat for our brain and that goes for all the other carbohydrate sources we could choose, including the ones we've discussed, or rice, potatoes or pasta that we've not. They are not mentioned just because there isn't that much else to say. There are grades of quality in everything – including rice, pasta and potatoes. The best option is always grow/make your own, that way you know it's fresh and you know what's in them! Obviously you can't grow your own rice, although the way climate change is progressing we may be able to grow rice in Scotland fairly soon! That said, if you do eat rice opt for basmati rice as it is higher in B vitamins – one of our 'Big 4' (more on those in chapter 8). You may not want to make your own pasta either but you can easily grow your own potatoes. They will grow really well in a large tub on the patio or at your back door. But again if you don't want to grow your own always go for organic or traditionally grown products from local producers. That may be tricky with rice – but as always buy the best quality you can afford.

Sugar

When we think of 'carbs' we usually think of bread, rice or potatoes – starchy foods. But carbs are also present in fruits and vegetables, a glass of milk, honey, jam or sugar.

In terms of quantity eaten, however, sugar is usually the winner. Sugar is another form of carbohydrate and gives us energy but it's a very poor substitute for some of the starch alternatives, or fruit and vegetables, because of its significant and far-reaching effects on our physical and mental well-being.

New research involving 70,000 women aged 50–79 shows that eating too much refined carbohydrates, such as those found in processed white bread, white rice and sugar, increases the risk of depression.

This makes sense. I've always been fascinated as to why there are more people on antidepressants in Greater Glasgow (where I live) and Greenock than other parts of Scotland. The link between depression and sugar may explain it – historically all the sugar arriving in Scotland came in via boats that docked in Greenock on the Clyde estuary. Scots took to sugar like ducks to water and, considering that nutrigenetics research has now demonstrated that our food preferences may be passed down the generations in DNA, the fact that our ancestors had access to abundant, cheap sugar means many are probably born with a 'sweet tooth'. The good news is that epigenetics research also shows we can change our gene expression by changing its environment. So with a bit of willpower we can minimise the impact of the sugar-rich diet of our ancestors.

White sugar has a dark history far beyond the mansions built by Scottish sugar barons off the backs of Caribbean slaves. Alexander the Great imported it from India around 325 BC, and it reached Egypt about 1,000 years later. Christopher Columbus brought sugar cane to the Americas. The sugar refining industry became big business and fuelled the African slave trade, many of whom were killed producing the sweet stuff Western nations had grown a taste for.

Sugar is bad for us plain and simple. It's highly addictive and leads to behavioural and mood disorders in later life. Studies mimicking the impact of drinking just one can of fizzy soda a day indicate changes to the prefrontal cortex. In case you're wondering, the prefrontal cortex is the front part of your brain responsible for planning, decision-making, complex thought, personality expression and moderating social behaviour.

Everything that you probably consider 'you' is made possible by the prefrontal cortex.

Fizzy drinks are a horror show when it comes to sugar intake. Since Japanese researchers worked out how to produce high fructose corn syrup (HFCS) from corn in the 1970s, it has found its way into just about everything, including processed food and fizzy drinks. This sweet syrup is one and a half times sweeter than table sugar and it's cheaper. I don't know about you but I don't know anyone who would eat 11 sugar cubes as a snack, but many of us do the equivalent of just that when we guzzle down a can of fizzy drink. That sugar is frying our brain and leading us down dark mental paths.

In another study published in 2010, the long-term effect of consuming too much sugar or sweeteners was investigated. Using adolescent rats (they never clean their room either by the way) it was concluded that when rats consumed too much sugar it triggered specific chronic depression and it was reported may increase susceptibility to psychiatric disorders. Again I'm not entirely sure what a rat suffering from a psychiatric disorder actually does, but the point is rats are used in these experiments because their physiology is remarkably similar to ours, so psycho rats usually also mean psycho humans!

And, before you reach for your sweetener instead – synthetic sweeteners are often worse! The artificial sweetener aspartame is made from the excrement of genetically modified bacteria. Yes, that little tablet you drop into your coffee with quiet satisfaction at having cut down on your sugar consumption is made of genetically modified E. coli poo!

Have you ever wondered why so many 'diet' products, processed food and fizzy drinks taste like shit – well now you know! Many nutritionists and health experts have branded aspartame 'the most dangerous foodstuff on the planet' and when you consider what it's made from it's easy to understand why.

I could literally list study after study, article after article, about the wide-ranging dangers of excessive sugar and synthetic sweeteners. If you want to read more follow the links in the reference section at the back of the book or simply Google it. But let's just cut to the chase. It's really not helping our waistline or our mental well-being and we need to cut our sugar intake right back. Period.

When it comes to sugar there is no such thing as quality sugar. Brown sugar is not better for you than white sugar; demerara won't save your brain cells. Caster sugar won't be any easier on your hips. It's all crap, so...

1. If you drink fizzy drinks – stop.

If that seems a little harsh then at least reduce the amount of fizzy juice you consume. Save it for a special occasion. When eating, drink water instead. Try sparkling mineral water if that makes it seem more appealing. Add a splash of fresh lemon and some fresh ginger if you're feeling really adventurous!

2. Cut back on all processed foods as they are loaded with sugar – especially 'low-fat' products. Remember 'low fat' usually means 'high sugar'.

3. Reduce the amount of sugar you add to food or drinks.

Dairy

When it comes to milk and its various by-products it's easy to forget that milk is actually the lactose secretions of a bovine mammal that's just had a baby. It is therefore baby cow grow fluid, just as breast milk is baby human growth fluid. It is designed for cows, not necessarily humans.

As a result, various studies have linked dairy products – milk, cheese, yoghurt etc. – to stimulating abnormal tissue growth in women, which leads to breast lumps, an overgrown uterus and fibroids, and can eventually lead to cancer. But dairy products don't just affect us girls; they are a key driver in giving men 'man boobs'.

Just a few decades ago nobody had heard of 2 per cent milk, half and half, or skinny milk. Our milk came in glass bottles with silver tops, not the different-coloured plastic caps we have today. There was only one type – full fat. Children up and down the country would fight for the cream that had settled at the top of the bottle to put on their porridge or cereal. Today the choice of milk is astonishing and most people opt for low-fat milk because that's what the government health officials advised us to do.

The problem, of course, is that the low-fat milk that dominates the dairy aisle in our supermarkets is tasteless white liquid stripped of nutrients and churned out by factory-farmed cows that may never see a blade of grass. Nine out of ten small, traditional dairy farms have gone out of business, replaced by massive dairy producers who operate very differently from the 'good guys' of yesterday. My neighbour is a local dairy farmer who is one of the few 'good guys' left in our area. He rotates his fields, his animals are raised on pasture, and yet he can't sell his milk to the supermarkets as they won't pay the price he needs just to cover his costs and break even. So instead he sells his 'naturally produced milk' to local artisan cheesemakers who then ship their premium products abroad or to upscale restaurants.

Unfortunately this is not an isolated story – the traditional farmers that are left can't get a decent price for their milk because the supermarkets often sell milk as a 'loss-leader'. This means they sell milk for less than it costs to buy it and a lot less than it costs to produce it to encourage people into the store, because they know that once someone is in the store they will invariably buy more than just the milk they came in for. Often a bottle of water will cost more than a bottle of milk! It's easy to see why farmers are protesting on the streets. Supermarket price wars have not only crippled local traditional dairies like my neighbour but it has reduced the quality of our milk, which now has far less omega-3 fatty acids, CLA and vitamin D compared to the full-fat, pasture-raised milk my granny had delivered every morning.

Scientists are now warning that sugar and refined carbohydrates are to blame for modern diseases like diabetes and heart disease – not saturated fat. And when you consider that full-fat milk only contains 4 per cent fat anyway it can hardly be considered a 'fatty food'. Besides it's the 4 per cent that contains much of the vital nutrients we need, such as vitamin D and omega-3.

So not only are we consuming cheap 'low-fat dairy' that has been stripped of most of its nutritional content but we are consuming far more of these 'empty' products than we used to. My granny had two pints of full-fat milk delivered to her door by the local 'milkman' each day and that would feed the whole family for the day. These days we guzzle down four-litre cartons, pour half a pint on our cereal in the morning, not to mention the grated cheese on top of spaghetti bolognese or pizza. Children's lunch boxes are chock-full of dairy – cheese strings or mini pots of fromage frais. But it's not just the Brits who love dairy. Americans are gobbling down a whopping 23 pounds of cheese every year.

The main reason is that it's cheap and supposedly good for us. If you were to ask 100 random people what was so great about dairy products, my guess is that at least 98 of those people would say 'calcium'. It's true that milk is a good source of calcium and when we were children it was a helpful addition to our diet as our bones were growing and developing. In UK schools all children were given a small bottle of milk to drink every day and that was certainly preferable to the fizzy juice or sugar-laden fruit juice that is in the lunch boxes of today's children. But, as adults, we really don't need that much calcium. We may need more in old age but there are much better sources than mass-produced low-fat milk. This mass-produced milk will almost certainly contain antibiotic residue passed into the milk from the cows. Those cows are also often given growth promoters and additional hormones to maximise milk production. When you buy non-organic milk at the local supermarket you are getting more than just calcium!

Besides, too much calcium competes with magnesium in the body because both these minerals compete for the same receptor sites in cells. If we consume too much calcium by eating lots of dairy and don't get enough magnesium, then the balance is knocked out of kilter and we end up deficient in magnesium (one of our 'Big 4').

With milk and other dairy products it's also about quality.

1. If you like milk, the best, most nutritional milk you can get is fresh unpasteurised milk from a traditional organic dairy. Unfortunately, because of European regulations it is very difficult to buy unpasteurised milk in the UK. It's also illegal in Scotland and the US.

So unless you fancy putting a cow in your garden...

2. Buy organic dairy products.

There are scientifically proven health and environmental benefits to drinking organic milk. Studies show that organic, whole and semi-skimmed milk has 68 per cent more beneficial omega-3 fatty acids, and higher levels of vitamin E and beta-carotene than non-organic milk. Dutch research has also shown that the incidence of eczema in infants fed on organic dairy products, and whose mothers also consumed organic dairy products, are 36 per cent lower than those who consume conventional dairy products. Even if you buy healthier organic dairy products use them sparingly, or eat dairy as a treat. There are far better ways of getting omega-3 and calcium without risking your health through eating vast amounts of dairy.

3. If eating yoghurt go for full-fat probiotic yoghurt. Full-fat cottage cheese (the low-fat variety was a firm favourite of dieters back in the 1970s) is also packed with tryptophan which helps promote serotonin production (the happy hormone).

4. If you only really drink milk because you are concerned about your calcium intake then consider switching to rice milk or almond milk – they are still high in calcium but without the lactose.

Fats and Oils

What we've been told as 'take to the bank' health advice has time and time again been proven incorrect. Fats and oils are another food category where prevailing wisdom has less to do with concrete health advice and more about money and who is pulling the commercial strings.

For decades we have been told that fat is bad for us. And yet the body needs fat – it is essential for health. Granted we don't need McDonald's Quarter-Pounder cheeseburgers, large fries and a full-fat smoothie every day, but we do need some fat.

What we assume as logical health advice is very often driven by commercial desires. Butter is basically milk, a touch of salt and very little else. It can't therefore be marked up that much. But what if we are told that animal fats such as butter and lard are bad for us and we should move away from these products towards the healthier oils and spreads. Add a few health claims on the packaging, fortified with some vitamins, and voilà – a new product that can be sold for considerably more than plain old butter.

Plus many of these new oils we are told to switch to, such as corn oil or maize oil, are actually just by-products of massive industries that want to find new and lucrative ways to sell their crop waste and convert it into new products that will further boost profits.

With fats and oils it's about quality and quantity. Don't believe all the hype about new products that might deliver certain health benefits. My personal favourite is the margarine that claims to lower cholesterol. In the TV advert we see a couple who are having their cholesterol checked. They switch to this new spread and start taking more exercise and lo and behold their cholesterol level falls. It's a miracle! Actually it's not – they started exercising more and got active – that's what probably lowered their cholesterol. It's not rocket science. Plus the cholesterol level that caused them both to panic in the first place was artificially inflated so that companies could sell us more products!

I've said it before and I'll say it again – it's a con.

1. Don't be afraid of butter and other animal fats – at least you know what's in them. But, use them sparingly.

2. Ideally buy organic butter. We are often put off blocks of butter because they get hard in the fridge which makes them difficult to spread. Consequently we end up using more. But my granny used to have a slab of butter in a butter dish that would sit outside the fridge all day. It was soft and easy to spread so we didn't use much.

3. Instead of corn oil, vegetable oil or maize oil, swap for high-quality olive oil, rapeseed oil or flaxseed, and hempseed oils that are naturally high in omega-3.

Locally produced rapeseed oil in the UK is good value for money but other brands can be more expensive. Coconut oil is also a good option as it is high in vitamin E and lauric acid (great for heart health) and has been proven effective in weight loss studies. Again, it can be more expensive and you probably don't want to fry your eggs in coconut oil but the health benefits speak for themselves, plus it also doubles up as a pretty effective body moisturiser! I often end up looking like a slug after covering my hair and body in coconut oil during a Friday night pamper session with a wee bottle of wine and a good film!

Water

Although not a food group, water is absolutely vital for health and yet the majority of us don't drink enough water.

A study conducted by sparkling water maker SodaStream in the UK revealed that only 23 per cent of those surveyed regularly drink the recommended two litres of water a day and over a quarter are unaware of the recommended daily water intake. Even more surprising was that over three million Brits said they thought soft drinks and energy drinks were better for them than water!

They're not. We need water – and tea, coffee or soft drinks don't count.

Of course, as with everything, quality also matters. Remember the bad halogens from earlier – fluoride is still added to drinking water in some countries including Ireland, the US and parts of Canada. About 70 per cent of Australians also have fluoride added to their drinking water, as do about 5.5 million Brits.

A recent report published by the Drinking Water Inspectorate (DWI) in the UK has found antidepressants and other pharmaceuticals such as bleomycin (chemotherapy drug) and diazepam in our drinking water, despite extensive purification treatments used by water companies. Published papers in science journals warn of the antibiotics and other drugs in our water.

When it comes to water:

1. Drink two litres a day. If you currently drink no water or very little water start by substituting whatever you drink with your meals for water. Have a water bottle with you at all times and drink regularly. That's the easiest way to ensure you drink enough. It can feel like a lot, but once you get used to it you will quickly feel the benefits. Drinking water helps flush out toxins and helps you to feel full without any calories so it's a win-win.

2. Buy a water filter. These don't have to be expensive. You can add a filter to your tap at home or simply buy a filter jug and fill it up every day and drink that.

3. Buy bottled water – although for most of us this is not necessary.

A Word on Organic

We've touched on organic food in various parts of the book but it's important to make a few points about organic food as a recap. Even today, organic food is often considered expensive and therefore only for 'posh shoppers' or it's only bought by hippy types!

As mentioned earlier, right up until the 1950s everything we ate was organically produced. The pesticides, insecticides and chemical fertilisers that are now commonplace in industrial food production were not yet commercially available, so organic food was the norm back then so normal that organic food was just called food because there wasn't anything else. Organic didn't require a label.

Today, however, 46 per cent of industrially grown food contains chemical pesticide residues and this figure is rising. In 2003 it was just 25 per cent and many of these chemical residues have been linked to developmental disorders, diabetes, mental health problems and cancer. In 2015 the International Agency for Research on Cancer (IARC) – the World Health Organization's cancer agency – classified glyphosate, the active ingredient in Roundup and the world's most widely used herbicide, as 'probably carcinogenic to humans'.

Chemical residue is hardly ever found in organic food. Organic producers are allowed to use eight pesticides but only when every other non-chemical approach has failed – but even then it's a far cry from the arsenal of 320 pesticides available to non-organic farmers. But it's not just chemicals added to the growing cycle – organic food can only use 45 food additives, derived from natural sources, compared to the thousands available to non-organic producers. Plus when you choose organic produce you have a bulletproof guarantee that what you've just added to your shopping basket is GM-free (genetic modification – more on that wolf in sheep's clothing shortly).

Outside of food quality, organic food production is also better for the environment, wildlife and employs higher animal welfare standards. Sure it may cost a little more but quality over quantity really does pay when it comes to food.

In 2011, Newcastle University researchers published a comprehensive meta-analysis of 343 studies (peer reviewed in the *British Journal of Nutrition*), 'The Case of Organic Fruits and Vegetables', which showed organic produce was at least 12 per cent more nutritious than non-organic fruit and vegetables (that's 12 per cent more vitamins without eating more calories – and no pesticides, herbicides or other toxins). Other studies have shown organic food is 40 per cent higher in antioxidants (vitamin C, vitamin E, carotenes (precursor to vitamin A)) than non-organic food. As mentioned earlier, research from Glasgow and Liverpool universities found organic dairy farm systems resulted in milk which has on average 68 per cent higher levels of omega-3.

It's worth pointing out, however, that I am specifically comparing organic produce to industrial food producers or the 'bad guys'. Small traditionally run farms often employ the same approach that is now considered 'organic' but unless they are certified as such they can't sell their goods as 'organic' goods.

For example, according to the Soil Association, the UK's leading organic certification body, organic farm animals:

- Must have access to fields (when weather and ground conditions permit) and are truly free range.
- Must have plenty of space – which helps to reduce stress and disease.
- Must be fed a diet that is as natural as possible and free from genetically modified organisms (GMOs).
- Must only be given drugs to treat an illness – the routine use of antibiotics is prohibited.
- Cannot be given hormones which make them grow more quickly or make them more productive.

- Must not be produced from cloned animals.

Organic arable farmers (those that grow crops) can only use a very limited number of chemicals – but only when other organic options fail. Most small traditional farmers or 'good guys', like my neighbour, already do most, if not all, of this and have always done so – but gaining official organic status is expensive and can take several years to achieve. The certification process is therefore often out of reach for the smaller producers. Anyway, why should traditional farmers have to pay thousands of pounds for a piece of paper saying they are doing things the way they've always done? Many of the 'old-school' guys see it as just another tax they need to pay for doing what their families have done for generations.

> *Easy Step:* If you know a local farmer and you know how they produce their food because you see them rotating crops and spreading manure not chemical fertiliser, consider approaching them to see if you can buy some products direct. If you don't know any local producers but you want to cut down on chemical residues and additives, then pay a little extra and buy organic.

Easy Step: If you live in the US check in with the Environmental Working Group (EWG) each year as they publish a 'Dirty Dozen' and 'Clean Fifteen' shopping guide. The EWG regularly test about 28,000 of the most popular fruits and vegetables to identify which are the most and least contaminated. Often buying organic isn't something we can do all the time either because of availability or cost, but as an absolute minimum you should avoid the 'Dirty Dozen' – 12 of the most contaminated fruits and vegetables in the US. Make it a priority to switch to organic for these products. The 'Clean Fifteen' are the 15 least contaminated fruits and vegetables and are the products you can most safely buy non-organic.

While there is no official UK or European version of these helpful lists, a Pesticide Action Network report published in 2013 showed that 20 of the 27 fruits and vegetables mentioned in the US lists also appeared in their analysis. The US lists are therefore a good indication of what to avoid and what's safer for UK and European consumers. In the UK the most contaminated fruits in order of contaminants were citrus fruit, pineapples, pears, apples, grapes, strawberries, peaches, nectarines and apricots. The most contaminated vegetables were tomatoes, parsnips, cucumber, carrots, lettuce, beans in a pod, peas in a pod, sweet potatoes, courgettes and marrows, and yams. If you eat any of these products regularly, then switch to organic.

'Food' to Avoid

Before we leave the food groups there are a couple of additional categories that we also need to cover – processed food and genetically modified foods.

Processed food

When we think of 'processed foods' we generally think of convenience ready meals and certainly that segment of the 'food' industry is thriving. More than three billion ready meals were eaten in Britain in 2014. They make up the biggest sector of the UK's £70 billion a year food budget.

But it's not just ready meals we need to be wary of. Processed food is food where the raw ingredients are processed in some way to turn them into something else. There is huge profit in ready meals for a number of reasons. For a start food manufacturers carry out little or no preparation of raw ingredients. It's cheaper and quicker to buy treated ingredients, mainly frozen or dried, from other companies. Meat, fish and vegetables are kept at sub-zero temperatures for months. But when the food is thawed and 'processed' into our microwave lasagne or fish pie it can be marketed as 'fresh'.

If you want fresh lasagne then I'm afraid you really are going to have to make it yourself – otherwise it (and all the other 'fresh' ready meals) is about as fresh as six-month-old bread. Plus many of these ready meals are laden with additives, fat, sugar and preservatives. Often they use the poorer-quality ingredients that can't be sold elsewhere but can easily be disguised in ready meals – think horsemeat beefburger scandal in the UK. Many of these food processing plants can churn out 250,000 portions a day using 70 different ingredients.

I remember when I worked for one of the largest food processors in the UK. I was charged with managing the Gordon Ramsay brand licence. Brand licensing means you produce food on behalf of the brand owner and benefit from using their name even though they don't actually produce the food. It was an exciting project to work on as Gordon wasn't just a celebrity chef in Scotland but was making quite a name for himself on the international stage.

For months I would fly to London and spend the day in Claridge's, one of London's top restaurants, to work with Gordon's executive chefs, coming up with (and testing) possible dishes that could be created as part of a new gastropub, 'posh nosh'-style range for Tesco and they tasted absolutely delicious. I would then take the recipes back to the product development team for them to replicate in the food factories. My job was to manage the expectations of the brand owner and the retailer, while ensuring a profit for the food processor, as we developed an exciting new 'ready to cook' Scottish food range for the supermarkets.

We tested the products in focus groups with resoundingly positive results. I managed the creative artwork for the new packaging which looked slick and upmarket – perfectly suited to the yummy food inside. 'Job done' as Gordon would say. Unfortunately, Tesco pushed for a lower price point and they insisted on a longer shelf life. Gordon and his team tinkered with the recipe but in the end they pulled out of the project because the quality of the initial ingredients had to drop to meet the price requirements and the number of additives and preservatives needed to meet the shelf life specification completely ruined the dish. In the end it tasted nothing like the amazing dish I'd sampled at the upmarket Mayfair eatery in London. Luckily Gordon and his team had enough integrity to ditch the project – refusing to put the Ramsay name on substandard products. However, not all celebrity chefs are the same. Sure, there are guys like Gordon Ramsay who truly care about what we are eating, but just because you see a celebrity photo on a product don't think for one second it is any better than the other processed tins, jars and packets on the shelf . . . and don't kid yourself into thinking this is what they eat at home – or what they serve in their restaurants. I can assure you they don't eat it at home and it is nothing like the spectacular dishes they serve in their restaurants!

Eating too much processed food changes our taste buds so we end up preferring this fake food to the real thing. Plus, studies in rats have shown that eating this processed junk food overrides our ability to appreciate when we are full – making overeating almost inevitable.

And if that wasn't bad enough, much of this highly processed food kills the good gut bacteria that protect us against obesity, heart disease, inflammatory bowel disease, autism and cancer. Studies conducted by Tim Spector, professor of genetic epidemiology at King's College London, could explain why some people put on weight while others don't, despite eating similar amounts of fat, sugar, protein and carbohydrates. After spending 10 days on a fast-food diet of McDonald's hamburgers, chips, chicken nuggets and Coca-Cola, the bacterial species in the gut reduced from 3,500 to 2,200 – 1,300 species were wiped out in just over a week on a heavily processed-food diet. This is catastrophic for mental and physical well-being because stomach flora play a crucial role in regulating metabolism and producing enzymes, alongside vitamins A and K, which help the body to absorb calcium and iron. Other studies have found that even mildly tweaking the balance of gut flora can alter brain chemistry and influence neural development and a wide range of behavioural phenomena, including emotional behaviour, pain perception and how we respond to stress. Simply put – when we kill off our gut bacteria by eating processed foods it makes us mad and fat! I've included a bunch of study links at the back of the book if you'd like to read more about this.

Remember, processed food includes everything we haven't cooked or made ourselves from raw ingredients, such as cook-in sauces, baked goods, breakfast cereals, ready meals and highly processed meat like hot dogs (to name just a few). Often we reach for these things because we are strapped for time or because we lack confidence in the kitchen. Take the packet mixes for example; we don't know how to make shepherd's pie so we buy a packet and follow the instructions…dice an onion and fry in a little oil, add beef or lamb mince and brown. Add a diced carrot and, according to the packet, you then need to add the dry ingredients from the packet mixed in water. Once thickened up simply add the mashed potato on the top and brown under a grill. But here's the trick – you were already making shepherd's pie – the packet was completely unnecessary. Instead of adding the processed ingredients probably full of additives and preservatives, simply add an organic stock cube, a little water and thicken up the gravy before adding the mashed potato. It's just as quick, cheaper (because you didn't buy the packet mix), tastier and minus all the processed ingredients.

Easy Step: Heavily processed foods make us mad and fat. Fact! So reduce these foods as much as possible or, better, completely eradicate them from your diet – at least until you are feeling better, and then have them now and again as a treat. If you do cave in you'd be far better eating a good old-fashioned portion of fish and chips from the local chippie than a ready meal, burger, takeaway pizza or even instant noodles. The fish and chips will probably be made from fresh, wild-caught cod or haddock and locally produced potatoes, plus it contains vitamins B6 and B12, vitamin C, iron, phosphorus, iodine and zinc. The average portion has 861 calories but if you half a portion and pile on the vegetables it's easy to reduce the meal down to less than 500 calories. Or even better skip the chips and just order a single fish with mushy peas.

Genetically modified food

As far as I'm concerned – and I'm not alone – genetically

modified food is a disaster for human health. Over the past few years a number of countries have completely banned genetically modified organisms (GMOs) and the pesticides that go along with them. My home country, Scotland, is the latest nation to ban this type of food technology, which is pretty ironic considering that it was the Scots that kick-started genetic modification when scientists from Edinburgh University produced 'Dolly the sheep' – the first cloned animal. Since then one of Scotland's most respected scientists has been sacked for speaking out on the dangers of genetic modification.

Árpád Pusztai is a world expert on plant lectins and has authored 270 papers and many books on the subject. He also spent 36 years as a leading research scientist at the Rowett Research Institute in Aberdeen, Scotland. In 1998 Dr Pusztai publicly announced his findings on a genetically modified potato study he had been working on – advising the British government and media that feeding GM food to rats had a negative effect on their stomach lining and immune system – causing major health problems. He said, 'If I had a choice, I would certainly not eat it and I find it very unfair to use our fellow citizens as guinea pigs.' Dr Pusztai was sacked as a result and publicly ridiculed – despite 21 European and US scientists supporting the findings of his work.

Pusztai is not alone. There have been numerous studies over the years that signal dangers associated with genetically modified food. Many leading scientists and academics believe we don't know enough about GMOs and safety tests have not gone far enough to prove these crops are safe for human consumption. They were only introduced to our food supply 20 years ago and there hasn't been enough widespread research on the effects of eating these so-called 'Frankenstein foods' nor have safe amounts been identified.

While I appreciate that our population growth means we need to feed more and more people, I don't believe genetic modification is the answer. Just look at the amount of food we currently waste because it's not pretty or doesn't make the supermarket grading system. Wouldn't we all be better to eat what we currently have access to before we go tinkering with nature too much? Plus I've visited one of the largest genetically modified food producers in the world – a monster of a company – and guess what: they don't even serve their own products in their own canteen. What does that say for the quality and safety of the products they are then pushing on the rest of the world? If you visit any major cigarette company, they have areas for people to smoke. Most cigarette company employees smoke – they know it's unhealthy and dangerous but at least they have the decency to smoke the product they are pushing on the world – but genetically modified food giants don't even do that!

Although my observational research on the use of GMOs is far from scientific, it scared me enough to be wary of eating these foods, or feeding them to my son. In 2008, I was working on a pork project for the Canadian government. I travelled up and down the country, visiting farms, meeting producers and understanding the supply chain from farm to fork. I met with a local rancher in Alberta, whose family had been producing pigs for four generations.

Unfortunately, the pork market in Canada at the time was heading south. Cheap US imports appealed to Canadian retailers who forced massive discounts on local pig producers. The far-reaching consequences of the global financial crisis in 2008 meant that shoppers everywhere were buying on price not quality. And this was crippling traditional Canadian farmers and paving the way for the cheap meat producers to gobble up market share. The traditional Canadian pig farmers, with high animal-welfare standards, sustainable feed regimes and outdoor-bred operations where pigs could live in a natural environment, free to roam and rootle around in the mud, could not compete with the US pork powerhouses who, at the time, caged their animals, docked their tails and fattened them up on an abnormal diet and chemical growth promoters. These animals lived a horrendous life – a life which was worlds away from the animals I visited on my trip to Alberta.

Due to lack of consumer demand for local premium products (which cost more) and supermarkets no longer willing to pay a fair price for his pork, he had to cut costs to keep the family ranch afloat – a farm that had been producing local Canadian pork for over a century. Normally the rancher grew his own feed but as the market dropped he was forced to sell off land and buy in cheaper, subsidised GM feed instead.

He showed me around the pens and fields where the animals lived. Many were sick. Some were dying. His vet bills were skyrocketing despite no disease or known pathogens present on his farm. 'I just don't understand it,' he told me. We both stood in tears looking at his sick animals. This was a man who truly cared for his livestock – and his wife would often feed piglets in their kitchen when their mothers were unable to nurse them. This guy was set to lose his herd, his ranch, his livelihood. The only thing that was different in the way he raised his pigs was the feed – GM feed. The local government was subsidising GM animal feed so he had taken up the offer. He told me, 'Switching their feed is the biggest mistake I've ever made.' I could see the pain in this man's eyes as he watched the sweat, hard work and care of his ancestors disappear before his eyes. He didn't want to be the one left with the legacy that he had failed the family tradition, ruined the business . . . and, more importantly, killed the animals they had worked so hard to care for. And yet that was exactly what was happening and there was nothing he could do about it because he didn't have the acreage to go back to growing his own grain.

What makes this all the more terrifying is that human anatomy is very similar to that of pigs. So this first-hand experience of the dangers of genetically modified food scared me enough to never touch the stuff again.

As well as my own experiences there are also many verified research studies warning of the hazards of GM food. One such study published in the *Food and Chemical Toxicology* journal in 2012 linked GMO corn and Roundup herbicide to rat tumours. After much controversy and criticism – many no doubt motivated by lobby groups – the study was retracted by its publisher on the grounds that the sample size of animals was too small to be considered effective. As mentioned earlier, in 2015 the World Health Organization classified glyphosate – the active ingredient in Roundup – as 'probably carcinogenic to humans'.

Roundup is the world's most widely used weedkiller and is mainly used on crops such as corn and soybeans, which are genetically modified to survive being sprayed with massive amounts of this herbicide. Roundup is manufactured by Monsanto, the largest genetically modified seed producer in the world.

GMO crops sprayed with Roundup are widely consumed all over the world. In the US 90 per cent of soybean and 80 per cent of corn is produced with Monsanto's GM seeds. Today, around 80 per cent of food in the US contains genetically modified ingredients. The most common GMOs are soy, cotton, canola, corn, sugar beets, papaya, alfalfa, squash and zucchini – or, as we refer to them in the UK, courgettes. These appear in processed foods and can be hidden in ingredients you wouldn't normally associate with GM crops, e.g. amino acids, aspartame, ascorbic acid, citric acid, sodium citrate, flavourings, high-fructose corn syrup, hydrolysed vegetable protein, xanthan gum, vitamins and yeast products. But this is not just a US problem.

In the UK most livestock, poultry and fish feed contains genetically modified ingredients including GM maize and soya. In fact, 85 per cent of all animal feed in the EU contains GM crops. The constant squeeze on farmers by the big retailers and processors has forced producers into seeking cheaper methods of producing meat. As GM animal feed is far cheaper than traditional animal feed, many farmers have been forced into using this feed for their animals. As of 2016, only one British food retailer guarantees a GM-free diet for livestock-supplying meat. That retailer is Waitrose – notoriously expensive and a store where most people who shop there don't even look at the prices. All other British food retailers, including Marks and Spencer – known for its quality food – use GM feed in their protein supply chains.

Of course, all this makes it pretty impossible to avoid GM – especially if you live in the US. So far, the UK and Europe are resisting the influence of GM but the companies behind GM are huge and incredibly powerful so it's hard to know how long we will be able to hold out against them. By far the biggest threat is the Transatlantic Trade and Investment Partnership (TTIP). TTIP is a series of trade negotiations being carried out in secret between the US and EU – similar to the TPP which has just been signed between the US and 12 Pacific Rim countries including Australia and New Zealand. It is a bilateral trade agreement that aims to reduce the regulatory barriers of trade for big business – including food safety. You might be reading this in the UK or Europe and be thinking, 'Oh, this GM stuff doesn't affect me.' Many European countries have banned GM foods; we don't raise animals in gigantic feedlots, pumping them with growth promoters and ridiculous amounts of antibiotics. Our crops are not grown using GM seeds. But here's what will happen if TTIP is agreed and passed into law. At the moment the US agribusinesses are complaining that they are at a competitive disadvantage because of EU food labelling laws. Our laws demand clear labelling on GM ingredients or how animals are raised. The US food giants might think this is unfair because once their products are allowed to be sold in Europe the labelling will put them at a commercial disadvantage. When given a choice between two products that may look the same the consumer will usually choose the one that is GM-free, adheres to strict animal welfare standards and is not chock-full of nasty toxins. What a shock! So the US will probably want to ban labelling so that the British and European consumer can't tell the two products apart. And to add insult to injury, they want to include a clause in the TTIP called the Investor-State Dispute Settlement (ISDS) which would allow them to sue countries that defy the labelling in an effort to differentiate their own traditionally produced, ethical and safe products from the mountain of crap that will flood the EU if TTIP goes ahead. Of course, farmers are in uproar about this in the UK and Europe but the farming communities are so small now no one cares – it's certainly not on the evening news.

If we don't stop this, by any means necessary, the sharp deterioration in public health caused by toxic and adulterated food imports may very well make it to the nightly news. Of course, by then it will be too late. There has been a significant decline in US health since GM was introduced there 20 years ago. The US is the 'sickest' Western nation and there are literally mountains of research pointing the finger at GM. If you Google 'GM links to illness and disease' there are almost 51 million results! Do we really want that virus spreading because of TTIP?

If you want to protect your food supply, and keep food labelling honest and transparent so that you can be informed about the quality, traceability and animal welfare standards of the food you buy to feed yourself and your family, then speak out against the TTIP – involve your local politicians, sign petitions and shout from the rooftops.

The best solution is to buy organic or buy your food from a local, trusted supplier and again steer clear of processed foods that are often laden with GM ingredients – none of which ever appear on the label.

They say we are what we eat and yet most of us think it's just a quaint old saying. It's not – it's absolutely stone cold fact. We are what we eat and if we continue to eat poor-quality, processed, chemical-ridden food, or agree to law changes that mean we can't tell the good food from the toxic, then we will continue to feel crap, look crap and stay fat and mad. Or we can realise that we are feeding more than just our belly – we are feeding our brain, our immune system and our emotions.

Part Four
Action Plan

'Only you can control your future.'

– Dr Seuss

Chapter 7: Take Your Power Back

'You can't just take an aspirin and sit around and have 12 donuts and think, "I took my aspirin so I'm not going to have a heart attack."
It's really important each person take personal responsibility for their health. You can't keep thinking that someone else is going to take care of it. You have to be part of the solution.'

— Corbin Bernsen

We need to completely rethink the way we think about food. Sure, food can be one of life's great pleasures – it's incredibly enjoyable and sometimes only a chicken korma or pizza will do. But instead of unconsciously reaching for the first thing that we can find or the quickest or easiest meal we can create, we need to ask ourselves what that food is going to do to our body and how it's going to make us feel.

Instead of doing what the experts say or the government guidelines stipulate, or even what our doctor may recommend, we need to question those 'facts' and make better choices for our health. We need to take our power back once and for all. Of course, I'm not saying that everything we are told is a lie, but a lot of the most common 'conventional wisdom' when it comes to food and health has been shown to be incorrect over time. And yet we don't upgrade our information or seek out new knowledge when it comes to our mental and physical well-being. Instead we accept blindly what we are told, eat the poor-quality or heavily processed food because it's easy, or we just keep taking the pills.

If you really don't want to be fat, mad or both any more then you need to seize back power and never relinquish it again.

Doctor Doctor: Get Tested

By now you will realise that the food you eat can heal or harm you and often you don't even know what's in the food you choose. If you are fat, mad or both, chances are you are already deficient in micronutrients or are consuming too much of certain products with their nasty side effects.

But what are you deficient in? Ideally the best first step is to make an appointment with your doctor and ask for some medical tests. Specifically ask your doctor to test for thyroid function and carry out a nutrient test on your blood. In particular, ask your doctor to check your magnesium, omega-3 and vitamin B levels, as these are three of the 'Big 4' for mental health (more on them in the next chapter). In addition, check your calcium and vitamin D levels because calcium, vitamin D and magnesium are interconnected and the proper balance of all three is essential.

Another important measure is to have your urine tested for HPHPA (bad bacteria levels) as this test will indicate whether you need more probiotics to keep your gut flora in balance (the fourth member of the 'Big 4'). It is also a good idea to check for food allergies as any allergic reaction in the body causes inflammation and a growing number of scientists now believe this may be a contributing factor in depression.

While many medics are still stuck on the theory that depression is caused by a chemical imbalance in the brain (a theory that has never been proven) and continue to prescribe SSRIs, a growing number of studies demonstrate the role of allergies and allergic reactions in mental illness. One study published in the *Journal of Affective Disorders* found that both depression and mania are associated with pro-inflammatory states and that cytokines increase when people are depressed. Cytokines are proteins that are produced when our immune system is fighting off a foreign substance – similar to when we have an infection or when we are allergic to something.

For many years as a small child my son suffered from asthma

and eczema. After that horrible allergic reaction while riding a pony on holiday I took him back to our NHS GP and asked for a range of tests to help us identify exactly what he was allergic to and what might be causing his health problems. My doctor said that he 'couldn't test for everything' and needed to know exactly what to test for. Not knowing what my son was allergic to or what nutrients he was deficient in I didn't know what to say, so we left the surgery without a blood test or appointment for allergy testing. Instead we were ushered out of the door with a prescription for an EpiPen should he have another severe allergic reaction, a prescription for Ventolin inhalers and steroid syrup!

As any mum will tell you, it's no fun watching your child suck on an inhaler or having to give them medicine every morning, so I decided to bite the bullet and take my son to a private clinic to test for his allergies. They took a sample of his hair and blood to test micronutrient levels and also conducted a biofeedback test on a medical device and then used kinesiology – where different foodstuffs were placed in his mouth to gauge the body's reaction. The results that came back shocked me. He was deficient in a whole bunch of micronutrients. And, he was also allergic to citrus and dairy! The freshly squeezed orange juice I prepared for him every morning, the milk on his cereal, macaroni and cheese for dinner, yoghurt in his lunch box – all foods that I thought were good and healthy for him but were actually the *source of his health problems*. You can imagine my guilt and anger that this had not been discovered earlier. My NHS doctor did very little to help other than provide pharmaceuticals to manage the symptoms. To be fair to the doctors, most are doing the very best they can. Often their hands are tied due to lack of funding for what are usually considered 'unnecessary tests' or they simply don't have access to up-to-date data and new evidence to help them heal their patients, especially when it comes to nutrition. It's as if doctors have been forced into being managers of health, controlling symptoms (with lucrative drugs from the pharmaceutical companies), rather than getting to the root cause of disease and actually healing the symptoms.

You need to put your foot down when you visit your doctor and state clearly the tests you want. If you live in the UK your GP or NHS doctor may try to resist conducting tests unless you meet certain criteria. With NHS budget constraints doctors are often under pressure to cut costs and told only to conduct tests where there is a 'need' for them. That means only for patients showing symptoms of a particular deficiency, imbalance or other criteria which merits spending money on laboratory tests.

Magnesium tests can be carried out on the NHS if you have symptoms of nausea, weakness or an irregular heartbeat. The criteria for testing vitamin B levels are light headedness, fatigue or symptoms of anaemia. Omega-3 tests can be carried out but you may find this harder to secure on the NHS. If your doctor initially says no, you need to stand your ground otherwise you won't get the tests done, or you will have to pay for them privately, so it's worth persevering or seeking an accommodating GP.

Be sure to remind your doctor that a few simple tests are going to be much cheaper in the long run if they mean you can come off expensive medication and prevent all the escalating health issues you are likely to endure if you don't take your power back now!

Coming off Antidepressants

You will need to have another conversation with your doctor if you are currently on antidepressants, but focus on securing the tests first. When making changes it's always best not to start changing too much at once, otherwise it can become overwhelming and you may just pack it all in! Once you know what your test results are and have started to make dietary changes to increase your nutrient intake and/or supplement your diet with essential minerals and vitamins, you will be in a much better 'head space' to then wean yourself off the medication.

Once you've started to make progress with your diet and

have increased your micronutrient level, it's time to reduce your dose of antidepressants if you are currently on them. When I raised this subject with my doctor he was unwilling to do it, but if you are following the guidelines in this book and vastly increasing your micronutrient intake as well as reducing toxins and stress levels in your life, there is no reason why your GP should not support your desire to get off these addictive drugs. And if he or she doesn't support you then you may want to consider finding another doctor who will.

For the most part antidepressants are supposed to 'tide people over' during times of bereavement, acute stress and chronic depression. But once on them, it's all too easy to stay on them because we are terrified of feeling the way we used to feel. Taking them becomes a habit, and it never crosses our mind that we could actually stop taking them, with guidance from our GP and feel better than we have in years.

Once you start eating a nutrient-rich diet or taking supplements that support proper brain function (more on that in the next two chapters) you will become less reliant on the antidepressants and can take down the dosage a little at a time. Many people are on 20mg per day so reducing by 2mg will minimise withdrawal symptoms. See how you get on and really tune into your body to see how you feel. If manageable, reduce your dose by another 2mg the following week and every week thereafter, until you are antidepressant free.

You may find that when you get down to the lower dosage level (under 10mg) that you experience some withdrawal symptoms. This is totally normal – these drugs are, after all, highly addictive. Your withdrawal symptoms may include sleep disruption, sickness and increased anxiety. If this happens you should increase the dose back up to where you last felt OK. Consider engaging in relaxation techniques (more on those in chapter 11) – and, when you feel ready, try reducing the dose again.

If you are taking tablets these can easily be halved or quartered. Capsules can be opened to remove some of the contents although your pharmacist may be able to help you with this. Liquid medicines can be easier to manage, either by taking smaller drops or by diluting the solution.

If you are taking multiple antidepressants it is usually best to come off them one at a time, reducing the original drug first. You will, however, definitely need your doctor's help in doing so, as reducing one drug may affect the impact of the others and create unwanted additional side effects. You must be very careful in this situation and take strict instructions from your GP on weaning yourself off the antidepressants.

Focus initially on improving your micronutrient level so you are in the best possible position – physically and mentally – to come off the drugs. And remember, reprogramming your behavioural patterns can be challenging, so it's best to do a little at a time. The good news is that behavioural change only takes 12 weeks to bed down and become the new 'norm'. You may have read shorter time frames in women's magazines or other 'quick fix' self-help books – but this isn't true. Psychologists have studied the length of time it takes to form new habits and the average is 66 days via something known as 'context dependent repetition'. For example, imagine that each time you get home in the evening you pour a glass of wine. When you first drink the wine upon getting home, a mental link is formed between the context (getting home) and your response to that context (drinking the wine). Each time you subsequently drink wine in response to getting home, this link strengthens, to the point that getting home comes to prompt you to drink wine automatically, without giving it much prior thought – thus a habit has formed. We all have numerous habits – especially around food. We need to break the bad ones and replace them with new healthier habits that will support our long-term physical and mental well-being.

One of those healthy daily habits may be taking essential supplements.

Chapter 8: Essential Supplements: 'The Big 4'

'I believe that you can, by taking some simple and inexpensive measures, lead a longer life and extend your years of well-being. My most important recommendation is that you take vitamins every day in optimum amounts to supplement the vitamins that you receive in your food.'

– Linus Pauling

We need to eat the correct balance of minerals and vitamins for our brain and metabolism to function properly. Often taking supplements can be seen as unnatural and that we should get our micronutrients from food. But even chimps take supplements when the food they normally eat is in short supply.

Researchers observed wild chimpanzees in the Budongo Forest eating and drinking from clay pits and termite mounds when their preferred snack of raffia tree leaves (full of important minerals for their diet) were no longer available. What I'm suggesting is no different. Ideally we should all improve our diet and do everything we can to reduce the toxins in our food. Increasing the quality of our food also increases our micronutrient intake. But if you are unsure what to eat or just want to be 'on the safe side' then adding supplements to your diet is a cheap and easy solution.

When it comes to being fat, mad or both – most people will be suffering from a deficiency in 'The Big 4'. They are:

- Magnesium
- Omega-3

- B vitamins
- Probiotics

Deficiency or imbalance in these 'Big 4' are so common and so widespread that even if you can't convince your doctor to give you the tests you ask for and don't want to pay for private tests, if you are currently part of the mad fat epidemic then take these four supplements and feel the difference. All four are very cheap to buy and readily available in health food stores or even your local supermarket.

Magnesium

Magnesium is the ultimate 'chill pill' and the wonder supplement everyone should have in their medicine cabinet – just like my granny did with her 'Milk of Magnesia' and Epsom salts. It is needed for more than 300 biochemical reactions in the body. It keeps our heartbeat steady, supports our immune system, maintains normal nerve and muscle function, regulates blood sugar levels, helps us sleep, reduces inflammation and prevents stress hormones from entering the brain. Although a vital nutrient for regulating metabolism (that controls weight) and mental health, a staggering 80 per cent of those eating a typical Western diet are deficient in magnesium. The RDA for an adult is between 320mg and 450mg per day, yet studies show most of us only consume 250mg – far lower than the amount our body needs for optimal physical and mental health.

Our ancestors would have consumed plenty of magnesium in seafood, organ meats and by drinking water straight from the stream or absorbed through the skin when swimming in the sea. But our diet and activities are very different today. Due to intensive farming soil is depleted of minerals, tap water has been stripped of magnesium during processing, and we've swapped the liver and onions or steak and kidney pie for processed foods containing little or no magnesium. Modern dwarf wheat strains which make up so much of the Western diet contain far less magnesium today than the einkorn wheat my granny ate. To make matters worse, millions of us regularly take antacids which further deplete magnesium in the body. As a result, we simply aren't consuming enough magnesium and it is a major contributing factor to the mad fat epidemic.

Doctors first became aware of magnesium as an essential mineral for mental health in 1968 when Warren Wacker MD and Alfred Parisi MD published their paper in *The New England Journal of Medicine*. Their research showed that magnesium deficiency could cause depression, psychosis, irritability, seizures, behavioural disturbances and headaches – all of which could be easily rectified by taking more magnesium.

Today, progressive medical doctors, such as Dr Carolyn Dean, are starting to treat patients with magnesium. In her book *The Magnesium Miracle* Dr Dean lists 56 different health conditions that research now indicates are associated with magnesium deficiencies including Alzheimer's, depression and diabetes.

Studies have also shown it combats everything from heart problems to osteoporosis, stroke and memory loss. It's the little white pill we should *all* be taking – especially if we are mad or fat. It is especially important if you also smoke. Magnesium has been proven to markedly improve lung function and studies show it helps to repair DNA in the lungs. This may go some way in explaining why my granddad lived to a ripe old age despite puffing away on full-strength cigarettes most of his life. His regular baths in Epsom salts and drinking Andrews liver salts probably extended his life without him even knowing it! Magnesium also helps combat respiratory disorders and is often used by progressive doctors to treat asthma and other conditions.

How magnesium interacts with other micronutrients

As mentioned in the 'Dairy' section in chapter 6, calcium competes with magnesium in the body as both minerals bind to the same membrane sites in cells. When we consume a lot of calcium and not enough magnesium this imbalance can kick-start a whole host of health problems including mental illness and obesity. Don't get me wrong, the body absolutely needs calcium (it's the fifth most common element in the body) but the secret to balancing these two minerals lies in understanding how they are absorbed, and monitoring how much of each you consume in your diet. The body tends to hold on to calcium by either storing it or recycling it, so even though we have a greater need for calcium it is harder for us to become deficient. That said, even if we have a plentiful supply of calcium it cannot be absorbed without magnesium and the body will draw magnesium from bones, organs and tissues to help balance the calcium. This can lead to a magnesium deficiency because, unlike calcium which is easily stored and recycled again and again, magnesium is used up or excreted and must be replenished on a daily basis. This is why so many of us are deficient in magnesium. We need regular top-ups in our diet and if we are not eating foods rich in this magic mineral every day, or taking supplements, then we soon run out.

The way that vitamins work is interconnected. How well one works depends on the amount of other vitamins and minerals in the body – so if you are deficient in one it can have a knock-on effect on the other. If you are not currently eating a diet full of dark leafy green vegetables, nuts, seeds, fish, beans, whole grains, avocados, bananas and dried fruit, but are regularly adding cream to your coffee, milk to your tea and on your breakfast cereal, cheese on pizza, parmesan on pasta and enjoy pots of yoghurt, then your calcium to magnesium ratio is probably out of kilter. If you are eating a typical Western diet there is a good chance you are consuming far more calcium than magnesium and you absolutely must take a supplement to balance this out. Another thing to consider is that calcium is often added to food products like breakfast cereals, fruit juices, crackers, antacids and many other processed foods. It is important to read the label carefully to see what foods are fortified with calcium.

Magnesium also competes with fluoride in the body and will

decrease absorption of fluoride when taken at the same time. This is good news for everyone who has fluoride added to their tap water because magnesium helps to minimise the negative impact of this bad halogen.

Magnesium supplements

The body typically absorbs between 20 per cent and 50 per cent of ingested magnesium so it is important you buy the best bioavailable supplement you can. Magnesium supplements are typically available as magnesium oxide, magnesium gluconate, magnesium chloride or magnesium citrate. Magnesium oxide tablets are the variety most frequently sold in supermarkets and pharmacies but they are poorly absorbed by the body. As a result you will need to take more tablets to ensure you are getting enough magnesium. It is often a false economy to purchase these cheaper tablets – plus, supermarket supplements often contain fillers and other unwanted ingredients and the elemental magnesium content can often be very low. By far the best supplement to take is magnesium citrate. It contains citric acid which is a mild laxative so a perfect choice for those of us with colon or rectal problems which are often associated with being overweight or obese.

Consider taking: 200mg of *magnesium citrate* – this is usually enough on top of a regular diet.

You can also use magnesium oil (magnesium chloride – not to be confused with the bad halogen chlorine) which is easily absorbed on the skin and also reasonably inexpensive to buy. Ten sprays of this usually deliver 150mg of magnesium or 43 per cent of your RDA.

Omega-3

Sixty per cent of the brain is made of fat. Forty per cent of this fat is long-chain polyunsaturated fatty acids (PUFAs) and DHA is the most abundant omega-3 fatty acid in the brain. Literally it's a no-brainer (if you'll pardon the pun) as to why omega-3 is so important for brain health. If omega-3 is a primary structural component in the brain then this fatty acid should be a key part of our diet if we want to stay sharp and free from depression or other mental health problems. It is widely accepted that almost all disease (including mental illness) starts with inflammation but omega-3 is a powerful anti-inflammatory so it makes perfect sense to ensure we get enough omega-3.

This may go a long way in explaining why omega-3 fatty acids have such a wide range of health benefits for those suffering from arthritis, asthma, depression, Alzheimer's, ADHD or heart problems. In fact, scientists have listed 61 health benefits from taking omega-3 fatty acids or ensuring we have enough in our diet.

A Japanese study published in the journal *Scientific Reports* showed that fish oil also aids weight loss. The researchers fed two groups of mice fatty food, with one group having fish oil added to the feed. The mice that ate the food with added fish oil gained significantly less weight and fat compared to the group without the fish oil. The scientists also measured energy burn and discovered the mice that ate the fish oil burned more calories. And that's not all – the study also showed that the omega-3 in the fish oil caused the mice to have lower insulin and fasting glucose levels which prevents diabetes. One of the primary measures for prediabetes and diabetes is a fasting blood glucose test. The test is done in the morning to test blood glucose levels before the person has eaten. The normal range for blood glucose is 70 to 100mg/dl – anything higher than this is referred to as prediabetes. Diabetes is typically diagnosed when fasting blood sugar levels are higher than 126mg/dl. This study is just one of many that shows the powerful healing properties of omega-3 fish oils and how they not only help us (and wee fat mice) lose weight but also fend off diabetes – a disorder which now affects one in ten Americans and almost four million people in the UK.

Omega-3 supplements

A recent YouGov study carried out for Fish is The Dish 'Feed Your Mind' campaign showed that 96 per cent of British adults don't know how much omega-3 they should be getting in one week and 73 per cent didn't know how much fish they should be eating. It's hardly surprising therefore that most of us are deficient in omega-3. This is also exacerbated because, as I've said several times, we are also eating far too much omega-6 and this imbalance is bad for our brain and body.

Just like magnesium, omega-3 gets used up pretty quickly in the body and needs to be replenished regularly in order to maintain balance and well-being. It is therefore essential that we eat a regular diet of oily fish such as: salmon, mackerel, rainbow trout, halibut, tuna, sardines and some seafood.

Omega-3 fatty acids are made up of three types – α-linolenic acid (ALA) (found in plant oils), eicosapentaenoic acid (EPA), and docosahexaenoic acid (DHA) (both commonly found in marine oils). These fatty acids protect the membrane of cell walls and influence the metabolism of cells. DHA (found in fish oils and algae) is the most important omega-3 for mental health as it improves communication between brain cells – hence the dietary focus on eating oily fish. Another great source of DHA is algae which is a good choice for vegetarians and vegans.

The RDA for long-chain fatty acids is 450mg per day but most of us consume around half this amount, with low-income families consuming considerably less. Of course, much of this has to do with the price of fish, or often the perceived price of fish, as we often assume we can't afford it. But fish such as mackerel, sardines or tinned tuna are still pretty cheap options.

Alternatively, omega-3 fish oil supplements, either in liquid form or capsules, cost pennies per day. The key consideration when choosing what supplement to buy is the concentration of EPA and DHA (the active ingredients for brain health). Even if you see 1000mg on the label this does not mean that amount of DHA and EPA is in the capsules. Look closely at the label to see how much of that 1000mg is made up of DHA and EPA.

Consider taking: A total of 500mg DHA and EPA per day – be sure to check the label to ensure your supplement contains 500mg of DHA and EPA not just 500mg of fish oil.

I have documented a list of published studies on omega-3 at the back of the book which not only provide scientific evidence that these fatty acids help to eradicate depression, but have been proven to prevent full-blown schizophrenia. There's some heart health, diabetes and weight loss studies too if you really want to do your homework!

B Vitamins

One of the most famous proponents of vitamin B therapy was Dr Abram Hoffer, a Canadian biochemist, medical doctor and psychiatrist who specialised in schizo-affective disorders during the 1950s. He was an addiction specialist and expert in niacin (vitamin B3) and, together with Bill W, founder of Alcoholics Anonymous, cured many people of alcoholism, drug addiction and mental health disorders such as schizophrenia and depression simply through administering high doses of B vitamins. He also worked alongside Nobel laureate Linus Pauling on orthomolecular medicine for cancer and treated thousands of patients using vitamin therapy.

Fast forward to the twenty-first century and B vitamins are now becoming more widely recognised in the scientific community as vital for brain function and the treatment of depression. Researchers at Kuopio University Hospital in Finland published a study in *BMC Psychiatry* which showed that people suffering from depression responded better to treatment if they had higher levels of vitamin B12 in their blood. Other studies have linked vitamin B12 deficiency with depression, anxiety and lethargy. Research published in the *International Journal of Geriatric Psychiatry* by a team of scientists from Oxford University found that daily supplements of folic acid, B6 and B12 were associated with a 30 per cent reduction in levels of homocysteine and improvements in a range of mental tests, including cognitive function and memory. Homocysteine is an amino acid which is produced as a waste by-product when we digest protein. If our homocysteine levels get too high it is associated with cerebrovascular disease (problems in blood supply to the brain), a drop in serotonin levels (the happy hormone) and increased instances of depression. Today, a growing number of scientists believe in the 'homocysteine depression hypothesis', which means they blame high levels of this amino acid waste product for causing depression in the first place. Needless to say it's incredibly important to keep this waste product in check by consuming enough folic acid, B6 and B12 – as these vitamins are the only way to remove this 'waste' from our bodies.

When I first learned of this it became abundantly clear to me why I felt so much sharper and the sky seemed bluer when I was pregnant and taking B vitamins as part of my prenatal routine. If I had only realised the connection back then I would have continued taking the B vitamins and could have saved myself years of misery after my son was born.

All of the B group vitamins affect brain function, mental sharpness and mood, and this is why B vitamins are part of the 'Big 4' – essential nutrients we must all take every day. Although it is possible to take each vitamin separately, you can also combine them all into what is known as a vitamin B complex supplement which includes:

- Thiamine (B1),
- Riboflavin (B2),
- Niacin (B3),
- Choline (B4),
- Pantothenic acid (B5),
- Pyridoxine (B6),
- Biotin (B7),

- Folic acid (B9) and
- Cobalamin (B12).

In order to hopefully prompt you into taking a vitamin B complex supplement every day, it may be useful to understand why these nutrients are so important and the impact they have on our brains. They are absolutely essential if you want to heal yourself and bid farewell to depression for good!

Thiamine (B1)

Thiamine is essential for proper brain energetics. If we are deficient our brain can't utilise glucose properly, leading to damaged DNA and degenerating neurons (dying nerve cells). It also plays a role in the body's absorption of foods containing carbohydrates. A thiamine deficiency can cause weakness, fatigue, psychosis and nerve damage in our brains. People who drink alcohol are more likely to be deficient in B1 so bear that in mind – the next time you pour a glass of wine consider whether you've had enough B1.

Foods rich in B1 include: sunflower seeds (this does not include sunflower oil as the vitamins are stripped out in processing), black beans, barley, dried peas, green peas, lentils, pork, fish and oats. Interestingly tea impairs B1 absorption – another thing to bear in mind as the average British person drinks 876 cups of tea each year!

Riboflavin (B2)

Riboflavin assists the body with growth and the development of red blood cells and, like B1, helps the body convert energy from carbohydrates. Studies show 27 per cent of adults are deficient in this vitamin.

Signs of deficiency include fatigue, cracked lips, sore throat and bloodshot eyes. How many of us have suffered from those symptoms, often putting it down to the weather or lack of sleep, and popped down to the chemist for lip balm?

Dietary sources include: dairy, meat, fish, eggs, mushrooms, almonds, leafy green vegetables and legumes such as peas, beans, lentils and peanuts.

Niacin (B3)

Niacin helps the body convert carbohydrates into glucose – the main source of fuel for our brain. It also helps the body use fats and proteins and is essential for a healthy liver, skin, hair, eyes and for optimal function of our immune system. Niacin improves circulation and has been shown to reduce inflammation (remember inflammation is a catalyst for most diseases so natural anti-inflammatories are very good for us!).

Interestingly, niacin also helps the body make various sex hormones, such as oestrogen and testosterone, and has been successfully used to naturally lower cholesterol levels for decades – long before statin drugs were created.

If you are deficient in niacin, symptoms include: indigestion, fatigue, mouth ulcers and depression. Even a slight deficiency can lead to these symptoms. Unfortunately, they are such common symptoms that many of us take them for granted and simply treat them with antacids and pharmaceutical gels. Most people suffer from mouth ulcers, with one in five people getting them regularly. Like everyone else I used to get them – but I don't any more because my body now gets enough niacin!

Foods containing niacin include: tuna, turkey, pork, liver, beef, portobello mushrooms, green peas, sunflower seeds and avocado.

Choline (B4)

We talked a little about the powerhouse nutrient choline in the egg section of chapter 6 and yet most of us haven't heard of it. Choline is really important for metabolism and the synthesis of molecules that are essential structural components of our cell membranes – allowing nutrients to enter and waste products to leave the cell. Like some of the other B vitamins, it also regulates homocysteine (remember that waste by-product produced when our cells metabolise protein). When we are deficient in choline symptoms include: muscle damage and abnormal deposits of fat in the liver causing non-alcoholic fatty liver disease (NAFLD). Around 80 per cent of obese people suffer from NAFLD, so if you are carrying more than a few extra pounds there is a good chance you have NAFLD and this could be partly due to a choline deficiency in your diet. Studies show that 90 per cent of us do not consume enough choline, so if you are mad, fat or both it is essential to top up on this vital nutrient.

As well as eggs, good sources of choline include: fish, meat, poultry and cruciferous vegetables like broccoli, cauliflower and cabbage. Unfortunately these vegetables have massively fallen out of fashion. When I was a child my granny would regularly make cauliflower and cheese sauce or cabbage soup, but trying to get a child to eat cabbage or broccoli today is no easy task! However, studies show that high intakes of cruciferous vegetables reduce our risk of lung cancer – probably another reason why my granddad lived so long despite his prolific smoking.

Pantothenic acid (B5)

Vitamin B5 is widely known to be beneficial in treating serious mental disorders, like chronic stress and anxiety. It has also been shown to alleviate symptoms of conditions like asthma, allergies, heart problems, respiratory disorders and hair loss. It performs a wide variety of functions including the production of neurotransmitters in our brain and the extraction of fats, proteins and other vital nutrients from our food. It reduces stress and anxiety by regulating the hormones which cause these conditions. Studies show that vitamin B5 reduces excessive production of cortisol – the stress hormone – that affects so many of us. Chronic stress from too much cortisol pumping through our veins causes an increased risk of anxiety and depression – so keeping this hormone at bay with regular doses of B5 is essential. Symptoms of a B5 deficiency include:

insomnia, anaemia, muscle cramps and burning foot syndrome (lack of feeling in your feet).

Foods high in B5 include: shiitake mushrooms, oily fish, eggs and gjetost cheese (a brown Norwegian cheese – perhaps another reason why folk in Norway don't get depressed as much as other nationalities).

Pyridoxine (B6)

Pyridoxine contains more than 100 enzymes needed for healthy protein metabolism. It recharges glutathione in our brains – a master antioxidant that gobbles up free radicals, heavy metals and other nasties. B6 is also important for red blood cell production, the nervous system and immune system, neurotransmitters in the brain and blood sugar regulation. When we are deficient in this nutrient it causes a lower immune system response, migraine headaches, chronic pain, depression and dermatitis (eczema). Considering that 35 million Americans suffer from eczema and 20 per cent of British children are now afflicted with this skin disorder, it really is about time we made sure we have enough B6.

As I mentioned earlier, my son's private medical tests came back showing a whole bunch of micronutrient deficiencies and vitamin B6 was one of them. The lack of pyridoxine in his diet, as well as other important nutrients, were the root cause of his eczema and caused horrible sores and scabs on his skin. Thankfully, once we knew what was going on it was incredibly easy to fix and he's never suffered from skin problems since.

Foods high in B6 include salmon, steak, whole grains, bananas, potatoes and beans.

Biotin (B7) (also known as vitamin H)

You may have seen biotin advertised on skincare ranges, shampoos and hair products, as it improves the keratin infrastructure of proteins which make up hair, skin and nails.

Like some of the other B vitamins, it helps our body to process energy and transport carbon dioxide from our cells.

Biotin can also help us with weight loss as it is involved in the metabolism of both sugar and fat, and makes it less likely to be stored as excess body fat. It aids the functioning of neurotransmitters in the brain that deal with cognitive function and our emotional well-being. And it also helps reduce blood homocysteine levels – that cell waste by-product again. Symptoms of biotin deficiency include: hair loss, nausea, muscle pains, anaemia, fatigue and depression.

Foods high in biotin include: liver, carrots, Swiss chard (one of the most popular vegetables in Mediterranean countries), almonds, walnuts, strawberries, raspberries, halibut, eggs, onions, cucumber and cauliflower.

Folic acid (B9)

Those of us with children will probably be aware of the benefits of taking folic acid during pregnancy to prevent miscarriage or birth defects such as spina bifida. Research also shows it is a useful nutrient for preventing colon and cervical cancer.

Mental health studies show that up to 50 per cent of people suffering from depression are deficient in vitamin B9. Even if you are just suffering from the fat side of the mad fat epidemic, 16 per cent of 'healthy' adults are also deficient in this nutrient as well as 19 per cent of teenage girls. Symptoms of deficiency include heart palpitations, weakness and behavioural disorders. A study carried out by the Iran University of Medical Sciences in 2009 showed that folic acid was effective in the acute phase of mania with patients suffering from bipolar disorder. In fact, I have a whole bunch of studies at the back of the book which support the claim that vitamin B9 deficiency is not only linked to bipolar disorder and depression, but can be used as an effective treatment for mental illness.

Foods high in folic acid include: lentils, dried beans and

peas, broccoli, Brussels sprouts, spinach, asparagus, citrus juice, cabbage and kale.

Cobalamin (B12)

Vitamin B12 is often called 'the energy vitamin'. We need it to make red blood cells, nerves, DNA, and carry out a host of other functions. Patrick J. Skerrett of Harvard Medical School said, 'Vitamin B12 deficiency can be sneaky and harmful.' This is because, unlike other water-soluble vitamins, B12 doesn't exit the body quickly in urine. It is stored in the liver, kidney and other body tissues, which means a deficiency may not show up for a number of years depending on your body's ability to absorb the nutrient and what you are eating in your diet. If you are deficient in B12 for a number of years it can cause irreversible brain damage. Certainly something to be avoided!

Like many vitamins, B12 can't be made in the body so we need to get it from food or supplements. The average adult requires at least 2.4 micrograms (mcg or μg) per day. People eating a strict vegetarian or vegan diet need to supplement with cobalamin otherwise they can encounter symptoms ranging from shortness of breath, irritability, fatigue, high blood pressure and depression.

But it isn't just human herbivores that are often deficient in B12, 20 per cent of people over 50 are lacking in this vital nutrient and recent studies from the US Framingham Study show that one in four adults in the US are deficient in cobalamin and almost half the American population is consuming less than they need. The Framingham Study is particularly interesting because it is a long-term study which began in 1948 to explore the cardiovascular health of residents in the small town of Framingham, Massachusetts, and is now on its third generation of participants with over 5,000 people already studied.

The reason that vegans and vegetarians are so susceptible to B12 deficiency is that this nutrient is not readily available in plants. It is found almost exclusively in animal tissues and good sources of B12 include liver, beef, lamb, venison, salmon, scallops, prawns, poultry and eggs.

Vitamin B supplements

As you can see, there are a lot of B vitamins, so taking them all may seem a little daunting. If you have the results of your blood tests then only take the supplements in the B vitamins that you are deficient in. If you've not had blood test results, then check that your diet contains plenty of the food rich in B vitamins.

> **Consider taking**: 100mg of each B vitamin and 400 micrograms (mcg or µg) of folic acid. Or take a B vitamin complex supplement which will contain all these and can help to plug any vitamin B gaps in your diet.

Probiotics

It may seem quite surprising but the bacteria in our gut can tell us a huge amount about our physical and mental health. Just like your fingerprint, the make-up of bacteria in the gut is unique to each of us. In fact, although we share around 99 per cent of our DNA with other people, we only have about 10 per cent of the gut bacteria in common. These tiny little microbes can influence whether or not we suffer from, or are saved from, conditions like heart disease, diabetes, depression and even obesity. As mentioned earlier in the book, there is now a strong scientific link between the health of the gut and the health of the brain. In fact, research linking probiotics to improved mental health goes back to the early 1900s.

Good bacteria in our gut increases levels of tryptophan, an amino acid that's required to produce serotonin in the brain – the happy hormone. Plus the different species of gut bacteria are essential for digestion so that our body can produce and absorb vitamins. Microbes also affect our mood. The enteric nervous system (ENS) has been referred to as our second brain and has up to 600 million neurons – equal to the number of neurons in the spinal cord. Emerging studies have shown that intestinal bacteria directly communicate with the central nervous system by way of nerve fibres and the immune system. Studies have shown that even minute doses of good bacteria in the gastrointestinal tract are capable of influencing neurotransmission in the hypothalamus – the part of our brain which regulates mood and emotions.

Probiotics reduce inflammation (a precursor of many diseases). They help us manage our weight by controlling the amount of energy we extract from food and by helping to regulate our blood sugar levels after eating. These amazing little organisms can literally determine whether we get sick or stay healthy and they have a major influence on our brains and waistlines.

A study published in the peer-reviewed journal *Obesity* is one of many studies confirming the link between balanced intestinal flora and weight loss. Researchers at Virginia Tech University discovered that good bacteria in the gut reduced the absorption of fat. Study participants were split into two groups and all followed a high-fat diet for four weeks. They were also given milkshakes to drink. One group had probiotics, including *Lactobacillus acidophilus* and *Bifidobacterium longum*, added to the shake, while the other group drank a placebo milkshake. Those who were taking the probiotic milkshake alongside their high-fat diet put on significantly less weight than those consuming the placebo milkshake.

Another study published in the *Journal of Clinical Investigation* in 2014 showed that mice fed probiotics didn't eat so much and had significantly reduced body fat and fatty liver, compared to the mice that did not receive probiotics. And in the *British Journal of Nutrition* a study reported that women who took a probiotic every day during a 12-week weight loss diet lost more weight than women who did not take the probiotic.

Probiotics also protect us against anxiety, memory problems and act like an antidepressant too. Researchers at the University College Cork have been studying the effects of probiotics on mental health and report that when study participants take probiotic capsules for just one month they experience less stress and anxiety and have lower levels of the stress hormone cortisol compared to the placebo group. Ted Dinan, head of psychiatry at the university who led the study, said, 'When they were given these bacteria they were less anxious and their ability to memorise material seemed to be enhanced.'

Even setting aside our mental health and weight issues for a moment, probiotics may also be our salvation in combating antibiotic resistance. A recent report from the European Centre for Disease Prevention and Control (ECDC) presents a stark warning on the increase in antibiotic-resistant bacteria in animals, food and us. In fact, 60 per cent of human gut bacteria are now resistant to antibiotics – partly due to the overuse of antibiotics in medicine and factory farming. Experts believe we are on the cusp of a public health disaster far greater than climate change or even nuclear war. And yet governments are still dragging their feet around animal and human antibiotic use.

The good news is that probiotics can help to minimise the antibiotic-resistant bacteria in our guts. By taking daily doses of probiotics we populate our gut with good bacteria and stop the bad bacteria multiplying out of control. The good bacteria in probiotics also help us to absorb vitamins – so we absolutely must ensure our gut has enough.

Probiotics are naturally present in certain yoghurts, fermented milk and kefir (a drink made from fermented milk), olives and sauerkraut – the stuff Germans eat with just about everything! But not everyone likes sauerkraut, olives and kefir – my son certainly won't touch any of them!

Consider taking: Two capsules containing three billion active cultures every day.

You could eat a probiotic yoghurt or yoghurt drink every day but they are far more expensive than standard yoghurt and significantly more expensive than a daily supplement which works out at just pennies a day. Probiotic supplements, available from your health food store, pharmacy or even your supermarket will usually contain at least four types of live cultures including *Lactobacillus* and *Bifidobacterium*. Some bottles contain capsules with 20 billion active cultures but again they are more expensive and frankly three billion live cultures is usually enough to plug any shortfall in your diet.

Magnesium, omega-3, B vitamins and probiotics are what I call the 'Big 4' for mental health. Even if you don't want to follow all of the advice in this book the very least you should do is ensure you have a daily dose of the 'Big 4'. I simply cannot stress this enough. If you are serious about taking your power back and regaining your physical and mental health then this is an absolute minimum.

Oh, and it's also worth noting that nobody has ever died from taking too many vitamins. Zero, zip, zilch, nada! On the other hand, thousands of people die each year from taking pharmaceutical drugs, taking the wrong drugs, or complications created from multiple drugs. So supplementing your diet with cheap, easily accessible micronutrients really is a no-brainer.

A Word on Recommended Daily Allowance (RDA)

The doses of micronutrients and probiotics that I'm suggesting may be different to the doses recommended on the bottles of supplements themselves.

There are several reasons for this.

First, we are specifically taking action to increase levels so that you can heal yourself if you are currently mad, fat or both.

Second, the doses on the bottle are usually based on outdated RDAs. There is now a growing body of research indicating that the RDAs stated by governments are simply too low and are designed to prevent deficiency rather than promote optimal health.

Plus, even the low RDAs don't take absorption rates into account. The companies that produce the supplements are legally required to list the content of the capsule or tablet in relation to the RDA. For example, the supplement may contain 100 per cent of the RDA or 80 per cent of the RDA but not all the active ingredient in the supplement will be absorbed by the body, so you will often have to take considerably more than you might imagine to ensure your body gets enough.

Ideally change your diet to include foods that are higher in the micronutrients you are deficient in – as identified by the nutrient and bacteria tests from your GP. Supplements are exactly that – meant to supplement your diet. The idea is that you take supplements to bridge the gap between where you are now, what you receive in food, and where you need to be. Pay attention to how you feel when you make the changes and let your body guide what you take.

Chapter 9: Additional Supplements to Consider

'Let food be thy medicine and medicine be thy food.'

– Hippocrates

Of course, there are many more essential micronutrients than the 'Big 4' but I've deliberately split them up so that you can better decide what's best for you. If you are curious about what I'm saying in this book and want to dip your toe in the water to see how you feel, then focus on ensuring an adequate daily intake of the 'Big 4'. If you are flat out committed to healing yourself, then you may also want to consider the various other additional supplements you could take.

Ideally, what you take or how you alter your diet to incorporate more micronutrients will be led by the results of your micronutrient tests. If not, then pay close attention to the symptoms of deficiency to help determine what may be missing in your diet.

Vitamin A and beta-carotene

Vitamin A was the very first vitamin to be officially named – hence it being awarded the first letter of the alphabet. Like vitamins C and E, vitamin A is an antioxidant and it is widely recognised for improving eye health, boosting the immune system, treating acne, preventing flu and treating other acute infections. It protects the body from the effects of toxic chemicals like those lurking in our household products and it has also been shown to help prevent the development of cancer – especially skin and lung cancer. Needless to say, it's an absolute must for smokers and sun worshippers to supplement their diet with vitamin A.

I've included vitamin A here because many of us are deficient in this micronutrient, not just because of the reduction in our food supply but because of a previously undiscovered genetic variation. Scientists at Newcastle University, led by Dr Lietz, have discovered that nearly 50 per cent of British women have a genetic variation which reduces their ability to produce sufficient amounts of vitamin A from beta-carotene (a precursor to retinol or vitamin A). The research also showed that all of the study volunteers consumed only about a third of their recommended daily intake of 'preformed' vitamin A – the form found in dairy, eggs and milk. As a result, Dr Lietz suggests that younger women are at particular risk because, 'Older generations tend to eat more eggs, milk and liver which are naturally rich in vitamin A whereas the health conscious youngsters on low-fat diets are relying heavily on the beta-carotene form of the nutrient.' In other words, we are not consuming enough of the right vitamin A and almost half of us have a genetic mutation which stops us from absorbing what we do get.

The news gets worse if you are overweight as further studies have shown that obesity causes a vitamin A deficiency. A Cornell University study published in *Scientific Reports* showed that obesity impairs the body's ability to use vitamin A appropriately and leads to deficiencies of the vitamin in major organs – even with adequate intake. The study also showed that when the weight was shed vitamin A levels returned to normal. Vitamin A deficiency can lead to chronic eye problems, diabetes, respiratory issues and abnormal immune response.

So, if you live in the UK there is a very good chance you are deficient in vitamin A. If you are carrying extra weight the organs in your body may be starved of this vital nutrient. Foods rich in vitamin A include: sweet potatoes, carrots, dark leafy greens, lettuce, apricots, bell peppers, fish, liver and tropical fruits.

Easy Step: Switch your morning juice to carrot juice – it tastes great mixed with freshly squeezed orange juice. Eat liver paté once or twice per week.

Or

Consider taking: 700 micrograms (mcg or µg) per day (RDA). Always read the label to check how much actual vitamin A is in the supplement.

Vitamin C (Also Known as Ascorbic Acid)

If vitamins were the Mafia then vitamin C would be the Don as it's the godfather of all antioxidants. It gobbles up those pesky free radicals we discussed in chapter 6. It increases the absorption of iron and chromium (an essential mineral found in various foods). In fact – as a side note – scientists have began testing chromium in large-scale trials as a treatment for mood disorders because small studies have shown it to be extremely effective in treating depression. I haven't listed chromium as a recommended supplement to take because if you are eating a regular diet and taking enough vitamin C then there should be no need for it. Just make sure you are eating enough broccoli, grape juice, whole grains and cereals, lean meat, organ meats, cheese, mushrooms, asparagus, green beans, potatoes, prunes, bananas, nuts, orange juice and even red wine – result! Some herbs and spices, such as black pepper and thyme, also add chromium to the diet, so when the cute waiter arrives at your table with the oversized pepper mill in restaurants, always say yes!

As for vitamin C, I can't stress enough how vital this antioxidant is for optimal physical and mental well-being. It plays an important role in producing collagen, carnitine and catecholamines. Collagen is the stuff that keeps our skin looking young. Carnitine helps our body turn fat into energy. Catecholamines are the hormones made by our adrenal glands, including dopamine, which is one of the hormones that regulates our mood and behaviour. Vitamin C is a powerhouse vitamin and we simply can't live without it.

Did you know that humans, monkeys and guinea pigs are the only mammals that can't produce their own vitamin C – every other animal on the planet can biologically whip up ascorbic acid in their bodies. Unfortunately for us (and monkeys and guinea pigs), a genetic mutation occurred that stopped us from producing it ourselves. Scientists have studied this extensively and shown that during times of stress animals produce up to 13 times the normal level of ascorbic acid to counteract the inflammation caused by the stress hormone cortisol pumping through their bodies. This helps explain why animals, unless they become injured, tend to remain pretty healthy until they reach old age, and non-vitamin C producing animals (like us) are more susceptible to disease. That in itself should be a pretty good indication of the value of taking a regular dose of vitamin C . . . but there is more.

Linus Pauling was an expert in quantum chemistry and biochemistry, and the only man in history to win the Nobel Prizetwice. Widely regarded as one of the brightest minds of the twentieth century, the *New Scientist* magazine ranked him as one of the 20 greatest scientists to ever live! Pauling coined the term 'orthomo-lecular medicine' and certainly I owe him a huge debt of grati-tude. It was my online discovery of orthomolecular medicine during my darkest days that sparked the beginning of my own recovery. His hypothesis appeared in 1969, stating that mental illness and disease are related to biochemical errors in the bodyand that vitamin therapy is a means of compensating for sucherrors. During his scientific career, alongside Scottish cancer expert Dr Ewan Cameron, Pauling cured terminal cancer patients using very high doses of vitamin C at 'The Vale of Leven Experiments'. He also wrote many books on vitamin C and advocated everyone should be taking high doses of this antioxidant – far higher than the recommended daily allowance set by governments.

Pauling himself took 12 000mg per day and lived until he was 93 years old, travelling internationally giving talks, lectures and interviews until his late 80s. To be honest, my son and I don't take that amount unless we feel a cold coming on – which is very rare. I also take more during periods of work stress and when travelling on long-haul flights, as this puts additional strain on the body. We safely take around 4000mg per day on top of what we consume in our diet. This is still significantly higher than the government RDA for vitamin C of just 60mg and probably goes some way in explaining why 30 per cent of the population are deficient in this vital antioxidant. Plus, of course, the fruits and vegetables we should get our vitamin C from have far lower quantities of the antioxidant today than just a few decades ago, so we need to compensate for the shortfall via supplements.

Vitamin C supplements are very safe to take as the body simply excretes what it doesn't use. One thing to bear in mind is that taken orally only 20 per cent is absorbed so if you take a 1000mg tablet you will only actually get 200mg. This is because most of it gets burned up in stomach acids and doesn't reach the liver. This is why my son and I take 4000mg – 20 per cent absorption still gives us 800mg to supplement our dietary intake.

There are other options, such as liposomal vitamin C sachets, which have very high absorption rates, but unless you are chronically ill regular ascorbic acid in high enough doses will do the job. Also, liposomal vitamin C is very expensive – currently only produced by a handful of labs who charge a fortune for their little sachets.

Serious deficiency in vitamin C is rare but many people are struggling to get by on very low levels. The elderly need more vitamin C as ageing inhibits absorption. Smokers also require more due to the oxidative stress caused by cigarette smoke. For everyone else there are some key signs that show you may not be consuming enough vitamin C – these include: dry and splitting hair, bruising easily, dry skin, gingivitis or bleeding gums and inability to ward off infections. Also, vitamin C is needed to heal wounds, so if you cut yourself and it's taking a while to heal it may be because you don't have enough vitamin C in your body. Instead of going to the shops to buy a mouthwash, expensive hair conditioner or more plasters to deal with these symptoms, buy some vitamin C instead.

Vitamin C is an essential supplement we all need to take to overcome the mad fat epidemic! It's cheap to buy and available in most supermarkets – although avoid the effervescent or chewable versions as they often contain aspartame and other nasty ingredients.

> **Consider taking:** 4000mg per day. Everyone's tolerance is different so it is often a case of trial and error until you find the amount that is right for you but 4000mg per day is a reasonable starting point. Even at 4000mg it is still far less than the 13 000mg produced naturally every day by many mammals or the 12 000mg taken by Pauling. Besides, if you take more than your body can tolerate the worst-case scenario is a short bout of diarrhoea, an upset stomach or a warm feeling on the skin (flushing) which quickly passes. Your urine might also turn orange for a day as your body flushes out the excess.

Vitamin D

Vitamin D didn't quite make it into the 'Big 4' but it was close. My goal is to ensure that you start to take action in regaining your mental health and waistline, so I've deliberately kept to the 'Big 4' as a manageable starting point. That said, vitamin D is also very important – especially for mental health. In the West vitamin D deficiency is soaring, with anywhere between 40 and 60 per cent of us not getting enough and in certain populations that rises to as much as 75 per cent!

Vitamin D is both a nutrient we eat and it is made by our body. When sunshine hits our skin it synthesises vitamin D from the cholesterol in our skin and is transported to the liver where it is converted into the hormone form. Unfortunately, climate change and our fear of skin cancer have meant that we don't get access to enough sunshine to keep our levels of vitamin D topped up.

Increased cloud cover in the northern hemisphere is definitely having an impact on our vitamin D levels. In parts of Scotland could cover has increased by 16 per cent in recent years, so we simply don't get the amount of sunlight we used to. Plus, when one sun does appear we immediately slap on sunscreen which prevents the synthesis of vitamin D in the body.

When I was a toddler growing up in Scotland in the early 1970s, summertime was so fleeting we spent every moment we could outside playing with friends. When it got too hot we made tents out of old blankets for shade, played in the close, or my dad would cool us down with the garden hose. I still have so many happy memories of squealing with delight as we played our own version of 'It's a Knockout' splashing around in the paddling pool and being chased by Dad with the hose. Our parents weren't out every five minutes lathering us up in Ambre Solaire factor 50 or P20. When we got a bit older we swam in the river and played in the forest for shade. Today we are so conscious of skin cancer many of us won't set foot outside in summer without some skin protection.

The problem is if we are low on cholesterol or sunshine then we don't get enough vitamin D. Plus to add insult to injury, we are no longer eating foods that are rich in vitamin D – like organ meat, eggs or full-fat milk. Effectively, it's a double whammy – we are not consuming enough or getting enough sunshine to allow our body to make it. As a result, we are seeing diseases like rickets, which virtually disappeared in the early twentieth century, becoming a public health concern in the UK.

But it's not just rickets; lack of vitamin D has a knock-on effect on how our body absorbs calcium and magnesium – one of our 'Big 4'. Vitamin D also activates genes that regulate the immune system and neurotransmitters – like serotonin, the happy hormone that affects brain function. This is why some people suffer from seasonal affective disorder (SAD) in the darker months – low vitamin D due to lack of sunshine interferes with serotonin levels in our brains. And with heavy sunscreen usage and a micronutrient-deficient diet some of us are turning summer into winter.

There are various studies linking low vitamin D levels to mental health problems (see references). If we don't get enough many of us get depressed – even those who do not normally suffer from mental health issues.

Vitamin D deficiency is also associated with obesity. Italian researchers at the University of Milan conducted a study on 400 overweight and obese people who were put on a low-calorie diet and then divided into three groups. One group took no vitamin D supplements, while the other two groups took either 25 000IU per month, or 100 000IU per month. After six months participants in both vitamin D groups had lost more weight than those who hadn't taken the supplements.

Another study published in the *American Journal of Clinical Nutrition* in 2014 showed that healthy levels of vitamin D were associated with weight loss in overweight women. In fact, the link between vitamin D and weight loss is slowly starting to gain interest in the scientific community with many more studies currently underway.

Foods high in vitamin D include oily fish, beef liver, cheese, mushrooms and egg yolks, so it is a good idea to eat more of these foods – especially in the winter months. Plus, when the sun comes out – get outside and soak some up! Obviously it's important to protect your skin but before you slather on your sunscreen spend a few minutes enjoying the midday sun on your bare skin before covering up or applying sunscreen. If you have darker skin, then you can enjoy a couple of hours without sunscreen.

Consider taking: 50 micrograms (2000IU) of vitamin D3 supplement per day. When taking vitamin D supplements it is absolutely essential to take the right kind. They come in two forms – D2 (ergocalciferol) and D3 (cholecalciferol). If you don't get much sun exposure or tend to slap on the sunscreen in summer, then it is vitamin D3 you should be taking as this is the type produced in the body when exposed to sunlight.

In the UK the RDA for vitamin D is just 5 micrograms (200IU) and 15 micrograms (600IU) per day in the US and Canada, but research shows this is grossly inadequate. A study published in 2014 titled 'A Statistical Error in the Estimation of the Recommended Dietary Allowance for Vitamin D' has created shock waves in the scientific community as researchers on both sides of the Atlantic have evidence to prove government guidelines are wrong by a factor of 10! We should be getting closer to 150 micrograms (6000IU) of vitamin D every day, not 15 micrograms (600IU). Taking an additional 50 micrograms (2000IU) as a daily supplement will help to top up your vitamin D level to ensure you get closer to the levels now recommended by scientists.

Easy Step: In the UK you can have your vitamin D tested inexpensively by the Birmingham NHS Trust. Visit http://www.vitamindtest.org.uk/index.html for more details. At the time of writing a single test costs £28 (discounts are available for multiple tests) and will be posted to you; simply follow the blood spot instructions and post back and you will have the results within seven days. This test is available to anyone in the UK.

Vitamin E

Most of us usually associate vitamin E with haircare and skin health as this antioxidant is widely promoted on personal care and cosmetic products. In fact, you will often find advice in the beauty tips section of glossy magazines recommending adding vitamin E capsules to your nightly moisturising regime. I snip the end off a capsule from time to time, adding it to coconut oil and moisturising around my eyes when I'm suffering from jet lag and look exhausted after a long-haul flight.

But vitamin E also plays a vital role in brain function and is an important nutrient for those struggling with their weight. A study from Oregon State University published in the *American Journal of Clinical Nutrition* in 2015 showed that obese people need more vitamin E than those who are not overweight. The double-blind study showed that the tissue from obese people reject intake of vitamin E because they already have enough fat. This is because vitamin E is a fat-soluble vitamin; in other words, it's stored by the body in fat so the body is tricked into thinking it has enough vitamin E because of the excess fat. If you are carrying extra weight you need to consume more vitamin E to ensure your body is getting enough.

As well as those carrying too much weight, people with decreased mental function and Alzheimer's disease are also more likely to have low levels of vitamin E. An international team of researchers published a study in *Neurobiology of Aging* which showed that Alzheimer's patients were 85 per cent less likely to have enough vitamin E and the findings suggested a direct link between oxidative stress in cognitive impairment and low levels of vitamin E.

As the name suggests, an antioxidant helps prevent oxidative stress in the brain and other parts of the body and, like vitamin C, vitamin E helps gobble up free radicals which cause cell damage. Vitamin E also boosts the immune system and helps to widen blood vessels and prevent blood from clotting.

Studies have also found that vitamin E helps to relieve period pain (dysmenorrhoea) and reduce PMS symptoms including anxiety, cravings and depression. In fact, one study showed that participants who took 500IU of vitamin E for two days before and three days after the start of their period experienced less symptoms than those who took the placebo. Every little helps if you tend to turn from Dr Jekyll into Ms Hyde every month!

A recent USDA study showed that 90 per cent of people eating a typical Western diet did not consume enough vitamin E, which is found in a range of foods including: dark leafy greens (spinach), broccoli, legumes, eggs, almonds, sunflower seeds, whole grains and olive oil.

> **Consider taking:** vitamin E supplements from a natural source. Dr Evan Shute, a physician recognised for over 30 years of work with vitamin E, suggests women should take 400IU per day. This is despite the fact that the Food Standards Agency (FSA) in the UK has set the recommended daily allowance at just 6IU.

Vitamin E exists in eight different types but the 'alpha' form is best as it is the preferred form of vitamin E transported and used by the liver. Also, if you do not get enough vitamin E from your food you must ensure you are taking a natural supplement. Synthetic vitamin E does not come from natural food sources and is usually made from petroleum products! Studies show that synthetic vitamin E is not as bioavailable as the natural form – meaning you need to take more pills. Also, many studies have shown that taking too much vitamin E can be bad for you – however, these studies often used synthetic vitamin E, not the natural alpha form. It's fairly obvious that consuming a by-product of the petrochemical industry is not going to be good for your health!

That said, by far the best way of getting more vitamin E is through eating more foods rich in this vital nutrient. Snack on a few almonds now and again – they are also a great source of calcium as well as vitamin E (ideally organic).

Selenium

Remember back in chapter 1 I asked the question 'So what happened in the 1980s?' in relation to the rise in obesity and mental illness? Well, another piece of the puzzle is that during the 1980s the selenium content in our food began to drop.

Selenium is a trace mineral found in soil and food. It is used by the body to regulate thyroid function and helps to make antioxidant enzymes which prevent cell damage. Like the other antioxidants we've covered (vitamins A, C and E), it keeps those nasty free radicals at bay. Some studies show that selenium can help prevent certain cancers and cardiovascular disease. It also protects the body from the poisonous effects of heavy metals and other toxins – like the 'bad halogens' and mercury vapour release from amalgam fillings when we chew.

As we covered in chapter 5, the thyroid assists in weight management by releasing hormones that control our metabolism. Therefore, nutrients that help our thyroid function properly, such as iodine and selenium, are essential for maintaining healthy weight. So if you're currently struggling with the fat part of the mad fat epidemic then you need to ensure you have enough selenium in your diet.

People who live in areas where there is very little selenium in the soil have a higher risk of becoming deficient. In the UK levels are very low as melting ice caps washed selenium from British soils 10,000 years ago and what little was left has been further depleted by intensive farming. Right up until the 1980s, most of the bread in the UK, a big part of our diet, was made with US wheat grown in soil naturally high in selenium. But when a major change in land use occurred during the 1980s many British farmers switched from growing barley to growing wheat (which was more profitable and had wider uses), so our selenium levels started to plummet. As a result, the British diet now only contains 50 per cent of the RDA of selenium which should be around 70 micrograms per day. Remember if the nutrient, in this case selenium, is not in the soil, it won't be in our wheat, fruits and vegetables, meat or milk we consume.

In fact, agricultural expert Professor Steve McGrath of Rothamsted Research (one of the oldest agricultural research institutions in the world) has called for small amounts of selenium to be added to fertiliser treating British wheat farms to increase our consumption of this important mineral.

Another key factor in British selenium deficiency is that by the end of the 1980s we were no longer eating offal, which is especially high in selenium.

But it's not just the fat part of the mad fat epidemic that selenium impacts. There are many studies linking selenium deficiency to mental health problems. A study conducted by the University of Otago and published in the prestigious *Journal of Nutrition* in 2014 showed a strong link between selenium concentration and depressive symptoms and negative mood. Co-author and study lead Dr Tamlin Conner is noted as saying, 'Our strongest finding was that those with the lowest selenium concentrations reported the most depressive symptoms. Although we did not test the physiological mechanisms, other research shows that oxidative damage to the brain and nervous system contributes to the development of depression. Adequate selenium intake is required for optimal antioxidant defences to protect body tissues from oxidative damage through glutathione peroxidise, which is a key antioxidant enzyme.'

Another review of five studies published in *Nutritional Neuroscience* showed that low-dietary selenium was clearly linked to poor mood and depression. And other studies have shown that selenium supplementation has proven effective for treating postnatal depression.

If you live in the US and are eating a lot of locally produced wheat-based products, you may not need a supplement as certain states in the US have reasonably high levels (although you may have GM to worry about instead). It's always a good idea to check your selenium levels just to be on the safe side – as even the smallest deficiency is enough to impact brain and thyroid function.

Foods naturally high in selenium include: Brazil nuts – with a whopping 1917 micrograms per 100 grams – just a small handful of Brazil nuts is more than plenty to ensure you get your daily allowance. Offal meat is also high in selenium. Oysters, tuna, wholewheat bread (if the wheat is grown in selenium-rich soil), fish and organic poultry are also good sources of this trace mineral.

Consider taking: 200 micrograms of selenium per day.

If you are unsure about how much selenium you are consuming then ask your GP for a test. However, if you live in the UK it's highly likely you will be deficient. A report compiled by Dr Alan Sneddon at the Rowett Institute of Nutrition and Health at the University of Aberdeen in 2012 states that the current average selenium intake in the UK is around 29–39 micrograms per day – half of the recommended daily allowance. The Rowett Institute report also states that, 'The human body can tolerate quite high levels of selenium without adverse effects on health. However high doses of over 900 micrograms per day can elicit toxic effects.'

Health store selenium supplements usually come in 200 microgram (µg) capsules, so unless you are going crazy on the Brazil nuts, or eating liver and kidneys for breakfast, lunch and dinner, it is safe to say a supplement of 200 micrograms is well below the upper tolerance level and safe to take. This is true despite it being higher than the RDA. Remember there is a growing body of evidence to suggest many of the accepted RDAs are set too low – sometimes far too low.

Iodine

Iodine was first discovered by the French chemist Bernard Courtois in 1811 when he was extracting sodium and potassium compounds from seaweed, which is chock-full of iodine. Like many scientific breakthroughs, Courtois came across iodine by accident when he added too much acid to his solution and a violet-coloured cloud emerged from his experiment. Iodine comes from the Greek word 'iodes' which means violet.

As covered earlier in chapter 5, iodine is a good halogen that is essential for thyroid function and also for general physical and mental health. Unfortunately, the bad halogens (fluoride, chlorine, bromine) are *much* more common. They are in our food supply, drinking water and environment, and they displace iodine in the body, effectively neutralising iodine's positive impact. As a result, most of us who eat a Western diet are now deficient. The scary part is that iodine deficiency is now accepted as the most common cause of preventable brain damage in the world!

Seaweed and sea vegetables have been used by the Chinese, Greeks, Romans, Egyptians, Polynesians and Celts for millennia as both food and medicine. The minerals and oils present in seaweed have long been used to recuperate from illness and ancient mariners called it 'sailor's cure' due to its high concentration of vitamins and vital nutrients.

Seaweed was a regular part of our diet right up until the Victorian era when it fell out of fashion due to the exciting new foods being brought back to the UK from around the world during the expansion of the British Empire. The invention of the steam engine also allowed greater distribution of these new foods.

Once again, giving up the old traditions for new foods maybe wasn't such a smart move. Seaweed and sea vegetables contain more vitamins, minerals and nutrients pound for pound than land plants and they are a cheap and healthy source of iodine. A study from the University of Glasgow published in the *British Journal of Nutrition* in 2014 not only highlighted that a lack of iodine in the UK population is now a prominent health issue, but the problem could be solved by taking Scottish seaweed in the form of a supplement. Study lead Dr Emilie Combet reported, 'This study shows that seaweed offers a way of addressing iodine insufficiency in a healthy, palatable way. Seaweed could easily be added to staple food groups with no adverse effects on taste. However, caution must be exercised – not all seaweeds are the same, with some containing too much iodine or heavy metals.'

The type of Scottish seaweed used in the study was *Ascophyllum nodosum*, part of the *Fucaceae* family of sea plants.

This is the same type that is widely used in sea kelp supplements in health food stores which has relatively low iodine levels. The women in the study took 0.5g of seaweed supplement per day – that's 350 micrograms of iodine.

Seaweed could also be the secret ingredient to losing weight too! Scientists at Newcastle University reported a compound found in common seaweed stops the body absorbing fat and that alginate found in sea kelp suppresses the digestion of fat in the gut. The study published in the peer-reviewed journal *Food Chemistry* showed that alginate found in seaweed reduced fat absorption by up to 75 per cent.

Crispy seaweed is sold in health food stores and many supermarkets but the taste is not to everyone's liking. Again, my son is not a big fan. Baked potatoes with their skin on, turkey, navy beans, tuna canned in oil, seafood and eggs are also good sources of iodine.

Consider taking: 350 micrograms of iodine. Look for seaweed or kelp supplements that are clearly labelled with the amount of iodine in each capsule. The easiest way to top up on your iodine without the fuss of cooking with seaweed is to take a supplement. However, buying seaweed or kelp supplements can be just as precarious as buying food. There's absolutely no point in taking a supplement each day if it is mass-produced and made from seaweed or kelp from polluted water.

There are some fantastic natural Scottish and Irish seaweed products available today, ranging from seaweed salt and seasoning (which we often use at home instead of table salt – it tastes great on home-made chips!), to skincare ranges, shampoos and soaps. These products are particularly good because our coastal waters are clean and the sea lochs boast a unique blend of minerals which the seaweed and kelp absorb. These products are now shipped all over the world.

> **Easy Step:** Use iodised salt instead of table salt in cooking.

Zinc

Although required in minute amounts, hence the term 'trace mineral', zinc is vital for human health. Even the slightest deficiency is potentially disastrous. This powerful antioxidant is found in every tissue in the body. As well as fighting destructive free radicals it helps to regulate our thyroid hormones (critical if you are trying to lose weight), supports our immune system and is essential for mental health. In fact, it has now been well established that zinc deficiency is common in several psychiatric disorders including depression.

Underactive thyroid (hypothyroidism) and overactive thyroid (hyperthyroidism) both result in zinc deficiencies and as zinc is required by the thyroid to convert T4 hormones into T3 hormones, when we are running low it can cause no end of problems. The way thyroid hormones work is pretty complicated but in simple terms T4 is a precursor to T3 and without adequate levels of T3 we start to feel fatigued, experience mood problems, suffer from depression or anxiety and struggle to lose weight. Too much T3 can result in heart palpitations, muscle weakness, insomnia and anxiety. The ideal balance of T4 to T3 should be around 17:1 and when this gets out of kilter we start to experience problems. If we are also deficient in iodine then it's a double whammy that can quickly lead to thyroid dysfunction and hormonal imbalance – making weight loss even harder. The balance of zinc and iodine intake is essential for thyroid function and, like so many of the micronutrients covered in this book, a deficiency in one can create a knock-on effect in our body's ability to produce or absorb another.

Obesity also often goes hand in hand with low zinc levels, so if you are carrying more than a few extra pounds you really need to be topping up. This is especially true if you enjoy a glass or two of wine or a few gin and tonics – alcohol further depletes zinc in the body.

Interestingly, zinc deficiency has also been linked to eating disorders like anorexia and bulimia – conditions that were previously thought to be 'all in the mind'. But like so many of these so-called psychological disorders, the root cause often lies in physiological problems – and in particular what we are eating and micronutrient deficiencies.

Dr William Gull first identified anorexia in 1873 and at the time patients were treated by force-feeding and surrounding them with people who could 'take control of their mental problems'. Today treatment is much the same, feed them, drug them and send them to see a shrink.

It wasn't until the 1970s that scientists began to spot the symptom similarities between those deficient in zinc and those suffering from eating disorders – a growing affliction which now affects millions of people living in the West. In fact, a recent National Eating Disorder report says about 30 million Americans are struggling with an eating disorder which they might not even be aware of! Claire Mysko, CEO of National Eating Disorders Association (NEDA), said, 'Countless individuals do not meet the clinical criteria to be diagnosed with an eating disorder, but are still struggling nonetheless. Not all symptoms are immediately apparent, especially if the cases have not had obvious physical effects.'

Today, progressive medics are successfully treating those suffering from eating disorders by increasing their zinc intake. If only this information had got into the hands of doctors treating Karen Carpenter and Lena Zavaroni then maybe these talented vocalists would still be with us today.

The highest concentration of zinc is found in meat and seafood. Needless to say, vegetarians and vegans are more likely to be deficient in zinc. The liver and onions, steak and kidney pie, and Cullen skink my grandparents ate were great sources of zinc and very different from the processed food we eat today. In fact, studies now show our zinc intake has declined over the past 60 years and a report from Professor John H. Beattie, Head of Micronutrients Group at the Rowett Institute of Nutrition at the University of Aberdeen, states we are consuming less zinc today than we were during rationing in the Second World War!

Like vitamin C, our bodies can't produce zinc so we need to get it from food or by taking supplements. Foods rich in zinc include: oysters with a whopping 74mg per serving, crab, lobster, beef, lamb, beans, whole grains and nuts. Dark cooking chocolate is also a great source of zinc so it's always good to add plenty when baking! The RDA for zinc varies from country to country but on average it is around 11mg. The upper safe limit is 25mg and studies show taking 25mg of zinc daily improves the immune system and helps minimise the symptoms of everyday colds and flu.

> **Consider taking:** 25mg of zinc citrate which is 61 per cent bioavailable. Remember, the dosage stated on the label doesn't usually equate to what your body will actually absorb. A 25mg supplement capsule will therefore deliver around 15mg of zinc which should be enough to keep you topped up and healthy.

Over two billion people suffer from mild zinc deficiencies and symptoms include lack of concentration and poor neurological function, weak immunity (always catching colds and infections), diarrhoea, allergies (runny nose, sneezing, hives etc.), poor night vision, acne, skin rashes or breakouts. In fact, I always know when I'm low on zinc as the skin on my fingers start, to peel slightly. If you are unsure about your zinc levels or recognise any of the symptoms, then it's best to ask your GP to run a test. If you are low then simply incorporate more zinc-rich foods into your diet or take a supplement.

Chlorella and Spirulina

We live in a world drowning in toxins. Our endless consumerism, technological advancement and pursuit of greater convenience, efficiency and speed means that toxins are everywhere – in the air we breathe, water we drink and food we eat. Air traffic, car exhausts, pesticides, herbicides, as well as the beauty creams, shampoos, washing powder, detergents, scented candles, mobile phones, cosmetics, even microwave radiation . . . the list is almost endless.

Companies manufacture trillions of pounds of chemicals each year and these are released into our atmosphere, our water and our environment. Arsenic, copper sulphates, lead and mercury are all found in inorganic pesticides and we are eating small amounts of these every single day if we don't buy organic food. But even if we do eat an all-organic diet, just breathing the air as we walk down the street exposes us to toxins. And, of course, let's not forget those amalgam fillings in our mouth releasing mercury vapours every time we chew.

Unless you live in an underground ice cavern in Antarctica or an untouched island in the Pacific you will definitely have ingested these toxins. If we don't keep them in check and find a way to neutralise them, they lodge themselves in our cells, soft tissues and muscles, and overwhelm our entire immune system. And if you're carrying extra weight your risks from these environmental toxins are even higher because there can be up to 100 times more toxins stored in our fat than in our blood. Over time these poisons lead to inflammation (the precursor to most diseases) and immune dysfunction.

A recent study by the Environmental Working Group (EWG) found the average person has over 91 toxic chemicals in their body. Most of these are known to be damaging to the brain and nervous system and some of them have already been linked to cancer.

Even pesticides such as organochlorides, which were banned in Western countries decades ago, still remain in the human body because they accumulate in the food chain and studies show that low levels of these chemicals are still found in the population today – especially in the West.

A study published in the journal *Environmental International* showed that individuals subjected to even low doses of organochloride pesticides over time are more likely to be diagnosed with mental health problems and weight gain compared to those not exposed to the chemicals. Other studies have also linked low dosage pesticide exposure to diabetes and heart problems.

But don't panic – a quick and easy way to get these toxins out of our bodies is to take chlorella and spirulina supplements.

Chlorella and spirulina are microalgae. Their molecular structure allows them to bond to heavy metals, chemicals and pesticides in your body, allowing them to be excreted naturally. They are powerful chelating agents that amazingly target the toxins while leaving other vital minerals intact. For example, chlorella does not bind with magnesium (one of our 'Big 4'), zinc and calcium, but it will bind to the likes of mercury, lead and arsenic. These smart little green pills are known as 'green foods' – and have been used as a food source and medicine for centuries.

Chlorella has existed on our planet for over 2.5 billion years; however, its powerful healing properties were not discovered until the late 1800s when it was first grown in Holland. In the 1950s the Japanese commercialised chlorella to boost food and nutrition and today it is the most popular food supplement in Japan with millions of people consuming it on a daily basis. Spirulina was a primary source of food for Aztecs and Mayans who used it to heal a variety of illnesses. It also has 12 times more protein than beef, making it a perfect dietary addition for vegetarians.

While chlorella and spirulina are biologically quite different they are both jam-packed with vitamins, minerals, amino acids and high levels of chlorophyll – the green pigment in plants that absorbs sunlight and uses its energy to synthesise carbohydrates from CO_2 and water. As you may remember from high school biology, this process is known as photosynthesis and forms the basis of almost all life on earth. Chlorella and spirulina are powerhouse nutrient-rich 'superfoods' that provide us with antioxidants and vital minerals, cleanse our bodies, help us to lose weight and fight diabetes. Studies have also shown that spirulina significantly increases the tumour-killing ability of natural killer cells in our body. Yes, these ancient green algae can kill cancer cells too!

In 2004 *Phytotherapy Research* published a study showing that chlorella suppressed weight gain in rats. Another study published in the *Journal of Medicinal Food* in 2008 showed that over a period of 16 weeks chlorella caused a noticeable loss in body fat, lowered LDL cholesterol (bad cholesterol) and blood sugar levels.

Chlorella has also been proven effective in reducing pain associated with fibromyalgia – a condition which is connected to both depression and obesity. One in fifty people living in the West now suffer from fibromyalgia and women are seven times more likely to get this disorder than men.

Detoxing our bodies is no longer the preserve of yummy mummy yoga types or New Age hippie vegans that live on juiced vegetables for a month at a time. It is something we all need to be doing – especially if we are mad and fat. Everyday toxins are stored in our fat and mess with our brain and immune system if we don't get rid of them.

I don't know about you but I struggle to do these January detox diets which always do the rounds on social media, and like most of us I usually cave in before the end of the month. Sipping hot water for weeks on end and swigging wheatgrass shots for breakfast is not my idea of fun – even if it is doing my body a power of good. The easiest way to tackle the toxin problem is to minimise exposure. That means eating organic food, especially for those foods that are laden with toxins (remember the 'Dirty Dozen' and 'Clean Fifteen' from chapter 6), and using chemical-free products in the home. Switch off your Wi-Fi at night, minimise your microwave use, and don't sleep with your mobile phone near your bed.

Beyond that, take 'green food' supplements in the form of chlorella and spirulina to filter out the rest.

Consider taking: 2000mg of chlorella and 2000mg of spirulina in tablet form. The RDA is between 3000mg and 10 000mg per day so 4000mg is well within the range.

You can buy these supplements in powdered form but when you add them to soups and drinks they don't taste fabulous. Tablets are a much more convenient option and cost just pennies a day – a tiny price to pay to rid your body of the harmful toxins we just can't avoid in the twenty-first century.

A Word on Herbs and Spices

Anyone who grows plants is probably aware of the health benefits of having some greenery around the house and flowers in the garden. They are great for producing oxygen and creating ambience. But did you know that plants can reduce stress, fight colds, cleanse your environment and even stop headaches? The humble houseplant can help us in so many ways but herbs can do so much more. Everyday culinary herbs can boost our mental health, fight depression, help us lose weight, reduce anxiety and even kill cancer cells! As Charlemagne once said, 'Herbs are the friend of the physician and the pride of cooks.'

My granny grew herbs on her windowsill and in the allotment. When I think of her I can still smell the geraniums and other plants and herbs she had around the house. Herbs should be a regular part of everyone's diet and no home, whether a studio flat in a high-rise apartment block or a mansion, should be without them as they are a cheap and easy way of adding vital nutrients to our diet.

You can buy the dried or fresh potted ones in the supermarkets but if you need a variety of herbs and eat them on a regular basis then the cost soon mounts up. Plus, just like the bags of salad, or pre-prepared fruits and vegetables in supermarkets, they will almost certainly be sprayed with pesticides and herbicides. As their leaves are so soft and permeable it is impossible to remove these toxins before adding them to your meals – even if you wash them. Also the dried ones can often be adulterated. A food study in 2015 revealed that 25 per cent of oregano tested in a range of shops in the UK and Ireland contained other ingredients. Food fraud is widespread with dried herbs – especially ones with a pungent odour where other ingredients can be added without affecting the look, smell or taste of the product.

Easy Step: Grow your own. You know they will be fresh without any nasty toxins. Growing herbs is easy, quick and the seeds cost pennies providing 30 plants for the same price of one plant bought in a shop. Sure, you will need some plant pots, trays and compost – but it still works out far cheaper and you get the pleasure of growing them yourself and the assurance they are clean and pesticide-free! Even if you can't be bothered planting seeds or don't have the time to wait for herbs to grow from scratch, you can buy store-bought culinary herbs and take cuttings – they will take root very quickly and speed up the growing process. Growing from cuttings is really simple and you can see a whole bunch of videos on YouTube showing you how to do it. Seriously, this is not rocket science!

Certain herbs will grow really quickly; others take up to 12 weeks until they are a good size. But once ready you can take as much or as little as you need and the plants will just keep growing. We use herbs every day at home, adding them to most meals, and I put them in my son's sandwiches for his school lunches. The powerful healing properties of eating just a few leaves each day can have a significant impact on our health.

Your must-have herb and spice supply

The best easy-to-grow herbs for weight loss and mental health are:

- Basil
- Coriander
- Rosemary
- Oregano
- Chives
- Sage
- Parsley
- Lavender
- Garlic, Ginger and Turmeric

All these herbs are really easy to grow on a windowsill. Even if you don't have a garden they can be grown indoors as long as they get sunshine and water. They will naturally fill a room with fragrance and add a splash of colour. Once ready, they can be added to just about any meal – from stir-fries, curries, soups, potatoes, rice, Italian tomato sauces, omelettes, sandwiches and much more. Even on that odd occasion when we do buy something pre-prepared in store, adding a sprinkling of fresh herbs can make something ordinary look and taste quite special and add a little home-made magic!

Basil

In India basil is known as the queen of herbs and for good reason. It fights inflammation (the precursor to most illnesses), protects cells and much more. Also known as 'holy basil' it has anti-anxiety effects and studies have found that the phytochemicals in basil play a role in lowering cortisol (the stress hormone). It has been used in India as a medicine for over 5,000 years and is a culinary staple in many traditional Indian dishes.

Studies show that increased cortisol levels and abdominal weight gain go hand in hand. This stress hormone has been shown to increase appetite and cause blood sugar abnormalities.

This amazing little herb is chock-full of magnesium and a great way of topping up one of the 'Big 4' in our diet. One hundred grams of basil also provides 105 per cent of our daily vitamin A needs, 30 per cent of our daily vitamin C and is packed with iron and vitamin B6. Basil is full of antioxidants which help keep those free radicals at bay.

Basil is one of the easiest herbs to grow at home. It grows like wildfire with hardly any care and attention. When I first started growing my own herbs I started with basil and planted the seeds in a few pots. Within just a few weeks I had so much of it I ended up giving bunches away to friends and making pesto so it wouldn't go to waste.

> ***Easy Step:*** If you do find you have too much then a great way of preserving basil is in pesto which you can easily freeze and use later. Simply whizz up the basil leaves, garlic, olive oil, black pepper, salt, parmesan cheese and pine nuts in the food processor and pop the mixture into an ice cube tray and store in the freezer. When you need a basil hit in your meals you can just take a cube or two from the freezer and add to your dish.

The smell of fresh basil growing in the house is wonderful and the luscious green leaves from growing your own surpass anything you can buy in the supermarket. It is a staple ingredient in tomato soups and sauces and can literally be added to just about anything – adding flavour and boosting those vital nutrients.

Coriander

Coriander (or cilantro) was a major part of ancient medicine. It was widely used by the Egyptians – coriander seeds were even found in the tomb of Ramses II at the famous Valley of the Kings site near Luxor. The Romans were also big fans of coriander and it was a key ingredient in one of their most popular drinks – posca. Posca was drunk by civilians and the Roman army to fend off disease. It contained a mix of sour wine, honey, coriander and water. In India coriander, known as dhaniya, meaning 'the rich one', was a staple of Ayurvedic medicine. It was also a firm favourite in ancient Greece where Hippocrates, the father of medicine, regularly used coriander in his medical practice.

Coriander contains chelating agents which bind to heavy metals (like mercury) and remove them from the body – in fact, studies show if it is taken with chlorella these two combined can remove up to 80 per cent of heavy metals from the body within just six weeks. If you still have metal amalgam fillings in your mouth then be sure to eat plenty of coriander (and chlorella).

Coriander is packed full of nutrients including vitamin B6, vitamin C, folates, vitamin A, vitamin K, iron and manganese.

Most overweight people struggle with digestive problems which can prevent weight loss. The volatile essential oils in coriander aid digestion and help us remove toxins from the body. Coriander has also been shown effective in treating Alzheimer's as it prevents neuron damage. Other studies show the volatile essential oil amyloid has cognitive-enhancing properties and improves memory! Coriander is known as the 'anti-diabetic plant' as it helps stimulate the secretion of insulin and lowers blood sugar. And it also helps to control the destructive free radicals we discussed earlier.

Next time you make soup, curry or a stir-fry add plenty of coriander – seeds, leaves or chopped-up stalks. Never underestimate how much of a positive impact this humble herb has on your brain and body. Plus, it's really tasty.

Rosemary

Rosemary is another amazing herb which has been quoted throughout history for its extraordinary properties. Tudors believed rosemary had hidden powers which enhanced memory, and in Shakespeare's *Hamlet* Ophelia states 'There's rosemary, that's for remembrance', and modern studies show the Bard's knowledge of this herb hundreds of years ago was remarkably astute. Researchers at Northumbria University have discovered that smelling rosemary can increase memory by up to 75 per cent. The magic ingredient in rosemary is called 1,8-cineole – not exactly a catchy name but this natural chemical has been shown to underpin memory.

But rosemary does more than boost our memory, it can improve mood, reduce inflammation, relieve pain, protect the immune system, stimulate circulation, detoxify the liver, help prevent premature ageing and heal skin conditions. It can also help us to lose weight!

A study conducted at the Nestlé Research Center – the food giant's study facility in Switzerland – showed that rosemary extract was able to inhibit weight gain and liver steatosis (fatty liver disease) in mice fed a high-fat diet. Researchers found that rosemary affects lipase in the body – an enzyme which breaks down fats. They discovered that rosemary extract may make you feel fuller by delaying the digestion of fats.

Nutritionally, rosemary is rich in dietary fibre which probably explains why we feel fuller when we eat this herb. It is also rich in vitamin A; just a few leaves of rosemary a day would almost meet the nutritional requirement for optimal vision. Fresh rosemary is also a good source of vitamin C and is very rich in B vitamins (part of your 'Big 4').

So if you want to remember everything you have read in this book, grow some rosemary, allow the aroma to permeate your home, and add it to your meals to help you feel fuller and aid weight loss.

Oregano

Oregano is a powerhouse herb for mental health and weight loss and helps with many other health issues. It supports the immune system, helps prevent and fight yeast infections, supports balanced blood sugar levels, fights swelling and promotes normal lipid levels (cholesterol). It has also been shown to clean as effectively as chlorine and is used by organic growers as an effective antimicrobial for disinfecting grapes and tomatoes. It has also shown interesting results in fighting cancer – killing breast, prostate and lung cancer cells in various studies.

The active ingredient in oregano is carvacrol, a chemical which can help us to lose weight. Animal studies have shown that carvacrol can prevent diet-induced obesity by modulating genes and reducing inflammation in fat tissues.

Oregano also stops fungal and yeast overgrowth (like candida) in the body. This is potentially important because a whole bunch of studies have linked weight gain to yeast overgrowth. Candida can cause stubborn fat deposits that are almost impossible to shake off – no matter how little we eat or how much exercise we do. Research conducted at Rice University in Texas shows that 70 per cent of all people are affected by candida, a systemic fungal infection that causes, among other things, sugar cravings. Like most fungi, candida feeds on sugar. When candida processes the sugar we eat, it lowers blood sugar levels and triggers the brain to tell us to eat more. So if you have a candida problem it may not be the psychological addiction to sugar that's the issue – it may be the candida itself as it feeds on the sugar and tells your brain to send it some more – thereby prompting us to gorge on carbohydrates and sugary treats.

Oregano is a powerful antifungal which kicks candida into touch before it can wreak havoc on our metabolism and waistlines. It has an impressive micronutrient profile – rich in dietary fibre, vitamin K, iron, vitamin A and manganese. It is also a good source of folates, B vitamins and vitamin C, so add it to your cooking. You can easily add oregano to most Mediterranean-style soups and sauces. It works well with tomatoes and even as a garnish on salads. I regularly use dried oregano in the same way most people use salt – this miraculous plant packs a punch and adds a huge amount of flavour from even the tiniest amount. Growing it on the kitchen windowsill fills the room with the smell of Tuscany, which sometimes tempts me into pouring a cheeky wee glass of Chianti while drying the herbs.

> ***Easy Step:*** If you have too many herbs, and this applies to all the herbs listed here, consider drying some. It's really easy to do – just cut a bunch and hang it up in a warm room until the leaves have dried. Then blitz them in the food processor and pop into an airtight jar.

When you consider how much a small jar of dried herbs cost in the supermarket (and there's no guarantee it's the real thing) then growing them yourself is a no-brainer. Again, oregano seeds cost pennies.

Chives

Chives are members of the onion family and are a good source of allicin. Allicin reduces levels of LDL (bad cholesterol) and increases levels of HDL (good cholesterol). Allicin also helps to reduce blood pressure – high blood pressure is a common symptom when we overeat, are stressed, or suffering from depression.

Chives also help to increase nutrient uptake in our gut – so we can absorb more of the vital vitamins and minerals we need to lose weight and fight depression. They are packed with micronutrient goodies – rich in vitamin C and vitamin A, both of which are powerful antioxidants.

You can easily add chives to mashed potatoes with a hint of garlic, or sprinkle a few chopped fresh chives on top of home-made soup or egg-fried basmati rice cooked in coconut oil, egg mayonnaise, or over the top of salads for a softer onion taste.

> ***Easy Step:*** Chives take longer to germinate from seeds so don't panic if they don't thrive like your basil. Don't give up; just keep them in a cool part of the house when germinating and they will emerge in their own good time!

Sage

Sage, also known as salvia, has been used for thousands of years as a powerful healing medicine. In medieval times it was known as 'toute bonne' meaning 'all is well'. In fact, the word salvia is derived from the Latin word *salvere* which means 'to be saved'. Stories of sage being used in religious ceremonies, mythology and witchcraft are also well known as it was classed as a sacred herb in ancient times.

Nowadays, it is a useful herb for physical and mental health due to its excellent antioxidant properties. It also helps prevent diabetes, reduces inflammation and protects brain cells. It helps to protect against the depletion of acetylcholine, an important neurotransmitter in the brain. You will remember we mentioned acetylcholine in the eggs section and that it was a neurotransmitter responsible for memory, mental clarity and connections between neurons. Just like the choline in eggs, sage helps to enhance acetylcholine levels in our brain, keeping us sharp and mentally balanced.

Nutritionally speaking, sage is packed with magnesium – one of our 'Big 4' – and just 100g provides 107 per cent of our

RDA. It is also a good source of vitamin A, vitamin C (hence its powerful antioxidant properties) as well as iron and calcium.

A meta-analysis of 43 previous studies published in *The Journal of Traditional and Complementary Medicine* in 2014 showed that the chemistry and medicinal property of sage can be used to help prevent and cure illnesses such as obesity, diabetes, depression, dementia, lupus, autism, heart disease and cancer.

Sage really is one of those 'all-rounders' we should always have in our kitchens. While most of us only use it for stuffing the Christmas or Thanksgiving turkey, it can easily be added to regular meals like meatballs and sausage meat. My granny used it all the time – adding it to gravy and bread for a bit of zing. I regularly add it to butternut squash soup or mashed potatoes, onions and a hint of garlic. It's yummy and super easy to grow.

Parsley

Parsley is the most popular herb on the planet. Charlemagne, the king who united most of Western Europe during the Middle Ages, was a huge fan of parsley and insisted it was planted in all royal estates. It has been used medicinally and religiously for thousands of years. Interestingly, the ancient Greeks believed parsley was too sacred to eat and the Romans adopted this custom only using it as a garnish. Maybe that's why parsley is still a popular garnish used in restaurants and food displays today.

But it's a waste just to use parsley to spruce up your presentation. It contains a plant compound called apigenin, a flavonoid which scientists now believe has the potential to treat depression, schizophrenia, Alzheimer's and Parkinson's. A study conducted at the D'Or Institute for Research and Education in Brazil and published in the *Advances in Regenerative Biology* journal showed that apigenin found in parsley, camomile and red peppers improves neuron formation and strengthens the connections between brain cells. Other studies have shown the volatile oils found in parsley – particularly myristicin – inhibits tumour formation in animals and helps prevent lung cancer.

The healing properties of parsley's volatile oils are classified as a 'chemoprotective food' that can neutralise carcinogens. Another study published in the *Journal of Traditional Chinese Medicine* showed that parsley has been effectively used as a treatment of gastrointestinal disorders, hypertension, cardiac disease and diabetes.

Parsley is packed with vitamin K – in fact, just half a cup of parsley provides a whopping 554 per cent of your recommended daily allowance. It is also a good source of vitamin C, vitamin A and folate. It is easy to grow at home but, like the chives, may take a few weeks before it germinates from seed. Once sprouted the seeds will soon grow leaves and before you know it you will have plenty of fresh parsley to add to potatoes, fish dishes, salads, dips and soups. It is great mixed with garlic and butter over roast vegetables. Don't be like the ancient Greeks and Romans: parsley is not just for decoration – it has powerful brain-boosting qualities and is great for detoxing the body.

Lavender

My granny always kept a wee pouch of dried lavender under her pillow as she said it helped her fall asleep. Again she was right as lavender is a mild sedative and the oil of lavender is used to make many different medicines.

Various studies have shown the powerful effect lavender has on brain activity – including nerve and mood responses. Inhaling lavender increases theta and alpha electrical signals in the brain and study participants who inhaled lavender were more active, relaxed and felt fresher than subjects who didn't. There are a number of studies showing lavender as an effective treatment for insomnia, anxiety, depression and fatigue.

A 2010 study published in the *International Clinical Pharmacology* compared lavender to lorazepam, a benzodiazepine (a type of psychoactive tranquilliser), and found for most of the test subjects lavender worked just as well as the drug.

While lavender has not been scientifically linked to weight

loss, getting adequate sleep has. In fact, a study published in the *Canadian Medical Association Journal* in 2011 showed that getting enough sleep radically improves the treatment of obesity and that when we don't get enough we are more likely to put on weight. With this in mind, using lavender to help us relax and get a better night's sleep is just as important as the antidepressant properties of this plant.

Lavender can be grown on a windowsill and then planted in the garden or potted in a window box or patio. Seeds will germinate in around two weeks but may take a while before the plant starts to look like lavender and flowers appear. Lavender prefers a poor soil and is perfect for dry rugged places in the garden.

If you grow or buy food-grade lavender then it can easily be added to meals. Most of us don't consider lavender as a foodstuff but it is regularly added to dishes in upscale restaurants and artisan food products. It's actually a member of the mint family and is also related to rosemary and sage. Why not try rubbing lavender on to lamb or duck, or even grinding it with sea salt to create lavender salt which can be added to butter for roasting potatoes and vegetables. It also tastes great in ice cream!

Even if you don't fancy cooking with lavender having it around the house and garden will fill your home with its relaxing aroma and you can dry the leaves and petals to use in the bath or for stuffing into your pillow just like my granny used to do.

Garlic, Ginger and Turmeric

I've included these three everyday food ingredients together because they really pack a punch in terms of nutrition, health and natural medicine. Garlic, ginger and turmeric are all powerful anti-inflammatories, antimicrobials and antibacterials that most of us have in our kitchen or can easily grow at home. Remember almost all disease starts with inflammation, so consuming more natural anti-inflammatories helps to protect our cells from damage. Antimicrobials prevent the spread of bacteria, fungi (like candida) and some viruses in our bodies. And, antibacterial substances can stop the development of bad bacteria in our gut. All three are incredibly useful when trying to fend off disease or the 'lurgy' as we say in Scotland. But these common foods don't just keep bugs away – they have been shown to improve our mental health and can even help us to lose weight!

Garlic

Bram Stoker famously wrote about the usefulness of garlic for fending off vampires in his classic novel *Dracula*. And although you may not need it for that purpose, garlic is a must-have ingredient in every kitchen.

The word comes from the old English word *garleac*, meaning 'spear leek', and just as the name suggests it cuts through disease and protects us from illness. In fact, garlic is one of the earliest documented plants used by humans for treating disease and maintaining health. It has been found in Egyptian pyramids and mentioned several times in the Bible. Ancient medical texts from Greece, Rome, China and India describe how it was used to treat a wide variety of illnesses – from lung disorders, parasites, flu, disinfecting wounds, joint disease and arthritis, cardiovascular diseases and much more. Our ancestors have used garlic for thousands of years to heal themselves and it's high time we did too.

It is packed with vitamin C and B6, manganese, selenium and a whole bunch of other antioxidants including allicin which is the source of garlic's antibacterial properties. Scientific research now proves our ancestors were right as garlic is effective for reducing blood pressure, cardiovascular disease, bad cholesterol (LDL), colds, flu and some cancers. It also improves our mental health by lowering homocysteine levels in the body. We've discussed this waste by-product several times (produced when we digest protein) and when levels get too high it creates problems in the blood supply to the brain, causes a drop in serotonin (the happy hormone) and increases depression. Garlic helps to keep homocysteine levels in check. Compounds in garlic also protect brain neurons from dying and increase circulation to the brain.

A 2006 study published in the *Journal of Nutrition* shows that, along with heart health, garlic can also help prevent Alzheimer's disease. The research indicated that garlic can not only curb the production of LDL cholesterol but lowers the production of a compound called -amyloid, which is seen in the development of Alzheimer's. By lowering -amyloid levels we lower the risk of Alzheimer's too.

Garlic has also been shown to help with weight loss – specifically because of the allicin. Laboratory tests have shown that rats given a high-sugar diet put on less weight if they were also given allicin – the compound found in garlic. Allicin is nature's way of protecting garlic from insects, fungi, bacteria and other pests which endanger the plant. It is also the compound that gives garlic such a pungent smell. Pretty useful if you want to chase away vampires or evil diseases!

Again, there are a bunch of peer-reviewed studies at the back of the book if you fancy some further reading on the healing properties of garlic. It should not be used just now and again in the odd pasta sauce or garlic bread side dish, we really must be using it as often as we can in the kitchen. I add it to just about everything – in varying amounts depending on the dish. It's great in soups, sauces, curries, stir-fries, pasta, salsa, pesto, mashed potatoes, roasted or sauteed with meat and fish, and it tastes yummy mixed into some soft cheese on top of oatcakes for a wee snack.

On those days when you are running about with no time to cook you could take a garlic oil supplement, and for those who hate the taste of garlic there are odourless versions in most health food stores. Setting aside the weight loss and mental health benefits, if you are prone to catching colds and flu during the winter season then adding more garlic to your diet is a must.

Ginger

Ginger originated in Asia. The Chinese and Indians used the root of the plant as a tonic to treat many common ailments. Apparently Confucius was never without ginger when he ate. It has been used for more than 5,000 years as a medicine and was first brought to the Mediterranean by traders in the first century. It was widely prescribed in ancient Greece and a famous Greek physician, working as a medic in the Roman army, wrote, 'Ginger warms and softens the stomach'.

Throughout history ginger has been used as an aphrodisiac, digestive aid and 'spiritual beverage' – which nowadays would be better known as a cocktail or alcoholic drink. It was also a pain reliever and the Japanese and Chinese have used it for millennia to ease joint and spinal pain as well as toothache. Thousands of years ago ginger was viewed as a healing gift from the gods and in the Quran ginger is described as a beverage of the holiest heavenly spirits.

In days gone by ginger was viewed as sacred and with good reason. The 'spiritual' qualities of this plant may have something to do with the benefits it has to memory, attention, neurotransmitter balance, brain ageing and inflammation, not to mention its curative impact on diabetes and obesity. Again, if you are in any doubt I have listed many studies at the back of the book.

Setting aside all the old folklore, ginger really packs a punch, not only in flavour and heat but in healing qualities. Ginger helps to stabilise our blood sugar, which is crucial if we are overweight, and it also fights the negative impact MSG has on our brain, helping to mitigate the effects of fast and processed foods.

Ginger tastes great in stir-fries, curries, desserts, home baking and in tea. If you are feeling bloated, tired, or are having an 'off day', infuse some fresh ginger in hot water for a refreshing pick-me-up.

Turmeric

Personally, I have a love-hate relationship with turmeric (also known as curcumin). It makes our chicken satay taste great but if you spill any on a light-coloured surface or clothing – it's a devil to get out. But it's the yellow pigments in turmeric that make it such a powerful medicine. Curcumin is one of nature's treasures and has been proven to fight cancer, obesity, mental health issues and much more. The yellow powder lurking in the back of your cupboard, used only for the occasional curry, has numerous hidden medicinal properties.

I first came across the healing power of turmeric when I visited India. It was my very own *Eat, Pray, Love* revelation and a holiday which changed my life for ever, prompting me to return to India time and time again. I was suffering from menstrual cramps and initially went to the spa for a massage but the girl mentioned pranic healing (more on that in chapter 10) and how it may be more effective at easing the pain – it was! We got talking and I explained that I worked in the food industry, so after she had finished the treatment she took me to the spa kitchen and introduced me to the chef who told me all about the healing ingredients he put in the meals. To traditional Indian chefs food is medicine (just like Hippocrates and the Greeks believed) and although didn't give me the exact recipes to his dishes (no chef worth his salt ever would), he did explain the curative properties of the spices he used. When I got home I researched it for myself and it turns out turmeric (or curcumin) has been used for centuries in Ayurvedic medicine to cure a myriad of diseases.

There are literally hundreds of modern scientific studies on curcumin but I have cherry-picked a few for you to review at the back of the book. Seriously, turmeric is like fairy dust when it comes to fighting disease. I couldn't quite believe it until I checked it out for myself.

It is a very powerful antioxidant and natural anti-inflammatory and one we should all be eating if we are mad, fat or both. Obesity creates a low-grade inflammation in the body that puts us at risk of developing other more serious diseases, like Type 2 diabetes, depression, heart disease and Alzheimer's. Turmeric can stop insulin resistance, high blood sugar, high cholesterol levels and other metabolic conditions caused by being overweight. It also reduces fat tissue growth in mice.

A study published in the journal *Phytotherapy Research* in 2013 proved to be a breakthrough as it showed remarkable outcomes in depressed individuals using curcumin. It was shown to target depression by promoting neurogenesis (the growth of nerve tissue), increasing levels of key neurotransmitters – serotonin, norepinephrine and dopamine (all important happy hormones) – and inhibiting inflammation. In fact, the study showed that curcumin was just as effective as taking Prozac!

We don't need to just use turmeric in curries and oriental dishes. I regularly add it to soup and sauces – even bread! It does make everything turn yellow but when you consider the healing power of turmeric it's a small price to pay for such medicinal properties. Just make sure you don't drop any on your white top!

You can also buy turmeric capsules in health food stores – but traditional Indian medics and holistic chefs swear that heating it first activates it further, so cooking with it is always best. It's also extra potent when mixed with ground coriander and/or cinnamon.

Action Plan Recap

We've covered a lot of ground in the last few chapters so this section is just to recap on what you need to remember and what you need to focus on to heal yourself.

1. You need to *rethink* how you think about food. Instead of just eating because you are hungry or in a hurry, start to consider the quality of the food you buy and eat. Is what you are about to eat feeding your brain, bones and body or just your boredom and your belly?

2. Make a conscious choice about the quality of the food you eat. Ideally you should know where your food comes from and how it's grown or produced. If you can, source locally produced, traditionally grown or farmed products that are higher in nutrients. If you can't or don't have the time or inclination, consider moving to products that are labelled organic – especially for fruits and vegetables that are highly contaminated as identified by the EWG's 'Dirty Dozen' and 'Clean Fifteen' shopping guides (or equivalent lists). Pay a little more for good-quality meat and cut down, or stop buying, cheap factory-farmed meat. By paying closer attention to what you buy you can ensure that the food you eat has significantly fewer toxins, chemical residues and higher animal welfare standards.

3. Visit your doctor and explain that you are unhappy with the state of your physical and mental health and well-being. You believe that part of the problem is a lack of micronutrients in your diet and would like to have some blood tests to establish if you are correct.

Specifically ask your doctor to test your:

- Thyroid function.
- Blood to measure your magnesium, omega-3 and vitamin B levels as these are three of the 'Big 4' for mental health.
- Magnesium, calcium and vitamin D levels because they are interconnected and the proper balance of all three is essential.
- Urine for HPHPA (bad bacteria levels) as this will indicate whether you need more probiotics to keep your gut flora in balance (the fourth in the 'Big 4').
- Reaction to various foods. Ideally check for food allergies as any allergic reaction in the body causes inflammation and inflammation is a contributing factor to depression.

4. Based on the results of your tests increase your dietary intake of the micronutrients you are deficient in or consider taking vitamin and mineral supplements to cover the shortfall between what you need and the micronutrients in the food you eat.

5. If you can't convince your doctor to give you the tests you require and don't want to pay for those tests privately, then at the very least consider supplementing your diet with the 'Big 4': magnesium in citrate form for easy absorption, omega-3, vitamin B complex, as well as daily probiotics.

6. Follow the 'Easy Steps' in the book as these really are easy, cheap and simple changes that can massively increase your micronutrient intake.

7. If you are also battling mental illness and want to come off your antidepressants, once you start to feel better as a result of the dietary changes and increase in your micronutrient levels, make another appointment with your doctor to discuss weaning yourself off antidepressants.

Chapter 10: Supporting Your Success

'Who looks outside, dreams; who looks inside, awakens.'

– Carl Jung

So far we've focused on food in our explanation for the mad fat epidemic. Specifically, how the modern Western diet is significantly deficient in micronutrients for various reasons and it is that lack of micronutrients that is having a profound knock-on effect on our physical and mental health. I've sought not to bamboozle you with too much science, but at the same time include enough so that you realise that what I'm saying is not just the idle ramblings of a crazy Scottish woman! I'm standing on the shoulders of scientific giants. I've also listed mountains of research, articles and links to additional information at the back of the book that substantiates all I've put forward in this book. To be honest, I don't expect you will read much – if any – of it, but I wanted to include it so you have the option to do further independent research if you want to.

I genuinely hope that you give it a go...Seriously, what have you got to lose? If you are currently fat, miserable and mad, then isn't it worth a shot?

Although we've focused on food it's also worth noting that healing yourself is not just about what you eat and the micronutrients you consume. It's also about the environment you live in. It's important to reduce the negative influences and increase the positive influences so you can support yourself as you make the transition from sick to healthier, miserable to happier, and fat to thinner.

Stop Looking at the Stars

As you prepare for change, stop looking outside for all the answers and instead start listening to your body. We have to stop worshipping youth and instead enjoy whatever stage we are at in life – whether 19 or 90! Stop wishing you looked like the stars you see in your favourite magazines – even the celebrities don't actually look like that in real life! Most have been tucked, plucked, sucked and Photoshopped to within an inch of their life! Learn to see through the fake world presented to us in women's magazines, TV shows and the cinema. It's not real and we have to come to terms with being ourselves instead of a poor imitation of the celebrities we see on screen and read about in the papers.

Look at some of the most powerful women in the world. Angela Merkel, Hillary Clinton, even Nicola Sturgeon who featured in *Vogue* in 2015 – these are not skinny women. Even the Spice Girls (the 1990s symbol of 'girl power') were voluptuous before becoming fashionistas with figures a mere shadow of their former, more healthy, 'normal'-looking selves. It amazes me why we always want to look like the supermodels instead of the 'real women' who are usually far better role models than the skeletal girls who starve themselves on a daily basis, or are born with unusually high metabolism or – worse – endure the trauma of cosmetic surgery to look the way they do. Also, most of the stars we gaze at with envy are incredibly wealthy and have an army of people looking after them. The women plastered over magazine covers all over the world are preened and pampered on a regular basis – they are not racing about in the morning, dropping the kids at school, sitting in the office all day, rushing home to make dinner and catching up on housework before collapsing into bed. No – they have their own chefs, personal trainers, regular facials, massage, aromatherapy, reflexology, manicures, pedicures and a whole host of other treatments which help to make them look the way they do . . . not to mention the odd tummy tuck, boob job and facelift.

Easy Step: Stop reading fashion and gossip magazines; just like food marketing, they are designed to fool you – creating the illusion that if you buy certain clothes or get your boobs done then you will look like your favourite celebrity. It's utter rubbish – especially as the celebrities they say we should aspire to don't even look like that in real life. Many of these already beautiful and slim women are even airbrushed and, to their credit, many will often come out and say so on social media. Not only is it a flat-out lie, but it sets an impossibly high standard that no one can reach. Why not use the money you spend on these magazines every month to buy supplements instead, or save the money and enjoy a spa session with your mad fat girlfriends as a treat. Trust me, it is far more rewarding than wasting your money looking at pictures of other people.

Love is the Best Medicine

R. D. Laing was a famous Scottish psychiatrist and philosopher working in the psychiatric hospitals of Glasgow during the 1950s. Through his work Laing noticed the psychiatrists hardly ever spoke to the patients they treated, and as an experiment he took 12 women and spent time talking to them about themselves and their lives. The women shared their experiences in a group forum, forging loving bonds with each other during the experiment, as well as receiving the attention of one-on-one therapy talking sessions with Laing. After just a few months all 12 women were well enough to leave hospital, as their symptoms of mental illness had completely disappeared. However, within 12 months Laing discovered all of them had returned to the hospital, suffering from the same symptoms they had been admitted with in the first place. Laing was curious as to why this had happened and began to investigate the relationships of these women. He studied how they and their families interacted with each other in private. Laing found that the roots of the women's madness originated in the home – it was the hostile and abusive relationships at home that were creating their madness. Of course, this meant that the doctors and nurses treating patients with ECT and other horrific treatments in order to make them well enough for them to return to their families were making a terrible mistake. As R. D. Laing so poignantly stated, 'Whether life is worth living depends on whether there is love in life.'

In 2010 neuroscientists at New York University's Langone Medical Center published a study in *Nature* backing up Laing's findings. They showed that oxytocin has a profound impact on how the brain processes social information. Oxytocin, often called the 'love hormone', is produced in the pituitary gland and stimulates feelings of love and satisfaction. Leading researcher Dr Froemke said, 'Our findings redefine oxytocin as something completely different from a "love drug" but more as an amplifier and suppressor of neural signals in the brain. We found that oxytocin turns up the volume of social information processed in the brain. This suggests it could be used to treat social anxiety, post-traumatic stress disorder, speech and language disorders, and even psychological issues stemming from child abuse.' Other researchers have linked increased secretion of oxytocin to less cardiovascular stress and stronger immune systems.

So what does this all mean? Basically, it means that even if you juice every morning, hit the gym before work, eat an all-organic diet and take supplements to keep your brain and body in tip-top condition, if you live in a toxic home environment or are constantly exposed to hostile relationships and never experience love, support and companionship, all the willpower and healthy eating in the world won't cure you. Love really is the best medicine.

There are many great ways to increase oxytocin levels in the body. Orgasms are high on the list, although if you have a toxic relationship they are probably few and far between. Of course, we don't always need someone else to help in that regard!

You can also boost your oxytocin levels by sharing a meal, talking to a friend, giving a gift, cuddling your pet, or giving and receiving hugs . . . lots and lots of hugs! Seriously, scientists have been studying this love hormone for years and have proven the more we produce the better we feel. So, get hugging! Take time to foster and maintain your friendships, and if a few of your friends are also mad and fat take the journey to health together, so you can support each other and bolster your supply of the love hormone. We are often conditioned to think of love in the context of a significant relationship or life partner, but we can experience love from a variety of sources – from family, friends or even pets. Of course, it's always wise to learn to love yourself too.

Learning to love yourself, or even accept yourself, is difficult – especially if you are mad and fat! But if you do not love yourself how on earth can you expect others to love you? I'm not talking about vanity, that superficial love of self when all you do is stand in front of a mirror preening or taking selfies. I'm talking about loving who you are on the inside, the sentient being who observes your body, listens to the chatter in your brain, and sees the world from a unique standpoint. We are not our bodies or our brains and many pioneering consciousness researchers, like Professor William Tiller at Stanford University, are making huge advances in this field of study. So if you don't like your body or the chatter inside your brain, you can change that – by taking your power back, following the nutritional guidelines in this book, and clearing out the clutter in your life.

'Clutter' can take many forms, from cheating partners, violent spouses, toxic friends, controlling family members and bad bosses through to actual physical clutter and stuff in your home. Of course, this isn't always easy and we often hang on to the things that hurt us the most – not just crap food and antidepressants! But if you truly want to heal yourself you have to take a stand and refuse to tolerate abuse or hostility in your life. If you have toxic friendships or family members that make you feel bad, limit the time you spend with them. You don't need to cut them out of your life completely, at least not straight away. Make the transition easier on you by simply avoiding their company for a while. When they phone or text for your help or want to meet up, just say you have other plans. You can easily limit contact without making a big deal out of it and causing a drama. This is likely to be easier on you – especially early on in your journey to reclaim your health.

Once you clear out the clutter and sort out your diet, life becomes easier and your health and happiness will improve considerably, which in turn will make it easier to really love who you are as a human being. Plus, it will give you more strength and courage to rid yourself of any other toxic influences in your life. Trust me, I've done it . . . and I haven't looked back.

Be Mindful of Your Emotional Triggers and Seek to Avoid Them

Minimising the triggers that bring on episodes of depression, anxiety, binge eating, cravings for sugar and carbohydrates, or reaching for the bottle, is an absolute must if we want to heal ourselves. These triggers can range from stress at work, revisiting trauma from our past, or from toxic relationships and the other 'clutter' we mentioned above.

The truth is, we all have a story to tell and most of us have experienced some sort of trauma in our lives, whether the death of a loved one, a failed marriage, family friction, redundancy or poor health. None of us are immune to the ups and downs of life – bad things still happen to good people. But when those challenges arise we stand a much better chance of riding the storm if our brain and body are functioning properly and are fully equipped to deal with whatever comes our way. This is why micronutrients are so important – they give us the strength to face whatever life decides to throw at us.

That said, it's important that you take the time to understand who or what kick-starts your emotional disturbances and do what you can to avoid those events or people. Of course, some of life's challenges, such as bereavement, can't be avoided and we simply have to cope the best way we can, but often – if we pay attention – we will see that certain people trigger our emotional decline. Think of yourself like an energy bank – and do an energy or mood audit against the people in your life. If you pay attention you may soon discover that you always end up leaving certain people feeling worse about the world and with less energy than you had when you met up with that person. Seek to minimise your time with people who drain you of energy and rob you of optimism about the future.

In situations where you really can't change what's occurred, you always have the choice regarding how you respond to those challenges and what you decide to make them mean. Changing our attitude towards problems and past events can make all the difference. And there's no point worrying about things we can't change either. As the serenity prayer reminds us:

> Grant me the serenity to accept what cannot be changed,
> The courage to change what can be changed,
> and the wisdom to know the difference.

Most of what we worry about never happens and yet that worrying can so easily kick-start a chain of chemical reactions inside your body that can seriously impact your health. My granny always used to say 'Worry gives a small thing a big shadow' and once again she was right. So let it go, and focus on the stuff you can change – including your physical and mental well-being.

Positive Interventions to Help You Succeed

Just as there are things that can trigger you into a sad or unhappy state, there are also things that can trigger or facilitate a positive mental state. These include, but are not limited to:

- Cooking as therapy
- Music
- Essential oils
- Good vibrations
- Reiki
- Mindfulness and meditation

Cooking as Therapy

One of the most positive changes we can make to support our long-term success is to cook our meals from scratch ourselves. Before you panic and throw the book across the room, I know the biggest reason we give for not cooking is time. This is especially true for mums who have to juggle a job while raising their children. As a result, we often resort to convenience foods because we don't have the time or inclination after a long day at work to cook from scratch. And as a single working mother myself I totally understand and relate to that. Grabbing a takeaway, a ready meal or just opening a jar of tomato sauce to heat and serve with pasta is a no-brainer sometimes. Nowadays almost everyone in the West eats prepared foods every day – from the quick cereal or granola bar at breakfast, shop-bought sandwiches and snack pots at lunch, and heat and serve tins, jars and plastic trays for dinner.

It's easy. But after everything you've read in this book I hope you realise that easy is not always good – and sometimes easy is contributing to the decline of our physical and mental health. So just hear me out...

It's true that in my granny's day women spent far more time cooking. Apparently in the 1960s women spent 100 minutes preparing the evening meal. In the 1980s that had dropped to 60 minutes, and today we spend just over 30 minutes making dinner. For single 20-somethings it can be far less – often a couple of minutes zapping something in the microwave. The reason for this is almost always time. I don't know about you, but my granny didn't work so it's easy to assume she had the time to cook. But is that really true?

Sure she didn't work in paid employment like many of us do today but she also didn't have a washer-dryer, a super-efficient vacuum cleaner, a fan-assisted electric oven, dishwasher, electric whisk, food processor, microwave, gas central heating, electric shower, disposable nappies or even quick and easy hair styling gadgets like curling tongs and straighteners. She had to beat the carpets and sweep the floor, wash the clothes in a twin-tub or by hand and hang them out on a line. There were no stain removers, so really dirty clothes, like terry-towelling nappies, needed to steep and she had to scrub the stains with a nailbrush. There was no tumble dryer or central heating radiators to dry clothes in her day. She had to clean the ashes from the fire, reset it, light it and keep it going all day. Dishes had to be washed and dried by hand. There was no non-stick convenience, so pots and baking trays with burnt-on food had to be cleaned three times a day after each meal. Shirts had to be starched and pressed with irons nowhere near as efficient as the ones we have today. Many natural fabrics had to be treated with special care; hand washed and dried flat. No chance of throwing on a pair of Lycra leggings and no-iron top for my granny. Clothes had to be mended, and she often made them herself on her old Singer sewing machine. Then of course she had to go shopping each day for food – cooking three square meals from scratch without the convenience of all the gadgets we have today. She didn't have easy wipe-down IKEA-style furniture so had to dust and polish all the wooden surfaces. Then there were the brass handles and knobs that needed buffing up with Brasso. Every day there was a long list of chores to do – which amounted to about the same time we now spend at work.

So, when we say we are too busy to cook – are we really that short on time, or are we just busy doing other things?

A recent Ofcom study showed that UK adults spend an average of eight hours and 41 minutes each day on media devices and almost four hours each day watching TV. Adults in the US spend an average of five hours and 31 minutes watching dvds each day and four hours 35 minutes watching TV. The average person has five social media accounts and spends one hour 40 minutes each day browsing these networks, scrolling on Facebook to see what everyone else is up to, sharing memes, looking at pictures of kittens and posting selfies!

Then there's the allure of gaming, like online bingo and Candy Crush – with over 45 million of us playing that game alone. While most of us assume video games are mainly played by spotty teenage boys in their bedrooms, a recent study published by the Internet Advertising Bureau showed that the majority of gamers are now women – not kids, not teenagers – us women!

We might all be working more but we spend countless hours each day frittering away our time on electronic gadgets. Now I'm not suggesting we all go on a Facebook-free diet, wean ourselves off television and stop watching videos so we have time to cook. What I am suggesting is that we can do both at the same time – I've been doing it for years without any withdrawal symptoms or sacrificing my favourite television shows.

Women are brilliant multitaskers. We can quickly move from one task to another and back again with ease. Being able to watch our favourite shows and chat with our friends on FaceTime or Skype while making quick and easy meals in the kitchen really is child's play.

Like millions of women I'm a sucker for soaps and I love *EastEnders* and *Coronation Street*. The thought of missing out on what Phil Mitchell is up to, or the next scheme Tracy Barlow is concocting, doesn't sit well with me. Working long hours and often travelling abroad on business can be challenging as up-to-date episodes are often not available in other countries. But with online catch-up, Netflix, TiVo and modern Sky boxes we can watch our favourite shows whenever we like and can also skip the adverts.

Because of my hectic work schedule Sundays are usually my preferred cooking day. And it really is therapy – I love it. I catch up on my soaps and other 'must-see' shows while pottering away in the kitchen making batches of nutritious food to add to the freezer. And I usually have a wee glass of wine while doing it!

When I first discovered the award-winning crime thriller *Breaking Bad*, long after it was first broadcast on AMC in the US, I was completely hooked and watched a series per cooking day. In fact, during my marathon session watching series one I cooked:

- A pot of tomato and basil soup
- A pot of carrot and coriander soup
- Roasted a fresh chicken and cut it up into portions
- Thai green curry sauce
- Italian Napoli sauce
- Bolognese sauce
- A batch of fishcakes
- Home-made bread
- Coconut-fried rice
- Mashed potatoes and blanched vegetables for the coming week

All while snapchatting what I was cooking, chatting to friends on Skype, and posting about how good *Breaking Bad* is on Facebook! Everything I make is then frozen in 'one meal' portion sizes by reusing the plastic trays from supermarkets and takeout meals. In fact, I have a cupboard full of plastic trays which I've reused time and time again – no need to go out and buy new fancy Tupperware sets.

It really is amazing how much food you can prepare in one day, or even one afternoon, which can then provide quick, easy and nutritious meals for the coming week or two. Just like shop-bought frozen meals, you simply take it out of the freezer the night before or in the morning before heading off to work, and when you get home all you need to do is heat and eat. A sprinkle of fresh herbs on top and voilà, a delicious, home-made, nutritious meal in the same time it takes to open a tin or jar!

Easy Step: Set aside an afternoon at the weekend and give this a go. Put on your favourite show and get cooking. You don't need to be a celebrity chef to cook. It's almost impossible to make a bad curry for example, and anyone can make soup. Often you don't even need a recipe – just put all the vegetables that are sitting in the bottom of your fridge in a pan with some stock, salt and pepper and simmer for a few hours to bring out the flavour. Experiment to see what you like. If you feel more comfortable with a recipe then you can find thousands of free recipes online.

Easy Step: Another time-saving tip is to start buying your groceries online or order from local companies that deliver. Making a list and buying only what you need helps you to save money and you will be less likely to succumb to the special offers and marketing tricks used to promote the foods we shouldn't be buying. The average person spends almost three hours shopping for food each week – this time could be better spent in the kitchen rather than walking around a store which is designed to tempt us. Home delivery from local vendors also saves carrying heavy shopping bags too!

Cooking is actually really relaxing and rewarding, especially if you cook Lockhart-style! Combine cooking with other things you love, TV, Facebook or chatting with friends and a nice glass of wine, and you'll soon find you look forward to your cooking day. Freezing meals frees you up from the 'I can't be bothered to cook' syndrome that pushes many of us to the ready meal aisle. It's cheaper and much, much more nutritious.

Of course, the cost of cooking will depend on what you currently have in your store cupboard. If you rarely cook then you may not have the herbs, spices and staple ingredients in your kitchen. The good news is that many of these ingredients are pretty cheap to buy, but consider spreading the cost and buy a couple of extra items each week – like spices, oils, vinegars etc. Growing your own herbs is super easy and will also save money.

Also, cook in large batches, as this always works out far cheaper than buying pre-prepared food. When I cook a large pot of soup, which provides many meals, the ingredients only cost a few pounds and home-made bread costs pennies. Similarly, a large pot of home-made Napoli sauce made from fresh and tinned tomatoes costs a fraction of the price of shop-bought pasta sauce. Consider buying cheaper cuts of meat for slow cooking – make tasty stews and cook whole chickens to portion up instead of buying expensive chicken breasts or steaks in the supermarket. Plus you can use the chicken bones to boil up and make delicious stock for your soups and other dishes.

A couple of years ago one of my friends took a keen interest in what I was writing about, and as an experiment we took one of her supermarket receipts and I bet her a bottle of wine she could save money by cooking from scratch with better-quality or organic ingredients. With a family of five to feed she had to buy several jars of sauce and packs of chicken breasts just to make one meal, umpteen boxes of cereal, loaves of bread etc. We went shopping together and bought lots of fresh and raw ingredients instead and got busy in the kitchen. Needless to say, at the end of the experiment I received a nice bottle of wine which we shared together. As I'd predicted, she saved around 20 per cent on her usual shopping bill *and* she was buying better-quality food. Today, she bakes her own bread, makes large pots of home-made soup, and a variety of sauces to feed her family – all while saving money. So much money in fact that after a year she was able to treat the whole family to a surprise holiday!

Like so many of us, my friend wasn't confident in the kitchen, hence her reliance on shop-bought sauces and packet mixes, but after seeing what she could save and how easy it was to increase the quality of the food she fed to her family she gave it a go. Her confidence has grown as she's realised that cooking isn't actually that complicated and she's never looked back.

The fact is that most of us eat pretty much the same collection of meals over and over again – family favourites. This means that you only really have to learn how to cook a handful of dishes and you are well on your way to better-quality food and better health. Home-made always tastes better, even when you're a novice cook. Plus you know what's in the food; there is no hidden fat, sugar, additives or preservatives to worry about.

OK – But what if I can't cook?

Long before I had the privilege of picking up tips from Gordon Ramsay and his executive chefs in a fancy London restaurant I knew very little, if anything, about cooking. Sure, I knew how to make pancakes, French toast and had my granny's favourite soup recipe but I hardly learned anything in school. But as US celebrity chef Julia Child once said, 'Cooking well doesn't mean cooking fancy.'

Unless your mum or granny cooked and you saw them cooking it's unlikely you will know where to start. School may have covered the basics but most people's experience of school cooking was a waste of time. As a result, most adults in the UK today don't know how to make a basic roux and I read a Sainsbury's survey of 934 people in 2013 which showed that one in three university students don't know how to boil an egg and 57 per cent can't cook vegetables.

Like most young women, my cooking skills didn't amount to very much. As a student I lived on tinned soup, beans on toast, instant noodles and cheese on toast. Then, I got my first serious boyfriend in my 20s and I knew I had to up my game. His friends were quite posh and dinner parties became the norm every other weekend as we all pretended to be grown-up and sophisticated. I knew it would be my turn soon but I made my excuses and desperately tried to figure out how to cook. I did this by watching *Ready Steady Cook* – a popular British TV show where guests and chefs had just 20 minutes to prepare a meal from scratch from a bunch of everyday ingredients. I would record it and then attempt to recreate it in the kitchen. I had to pause and rewind a lot but, surprisingly, with a bit of practice I got to understand what ingredients worked well together and basic flavour profiles. Within a matter of weeks I felt confident enough to take my turn with the dinner party – and to my surprise it was a roaring success. Little did they know I had just newly figured out how to cook from watching daytime TV, although I did top up their wine glasses regularly as a backup plan – so even if they thought the food wasn't great they had a good time anyway!

Seriously, if I can do it – anyone can do it. Even my teenage son can rustle up a few tasty dishes, so there really is no excuse. Most of us will never cook like the celebrity chefs but it doesn't matter. More often than not the same meal doesn't taste the same twice – but that doesn't matter either, so long as all the right healthy ingredients are in there, your mind and body will benefit from it and you will learn from the ongoing process of cooking. The best cooks improvise – and you should too.

There are literally millions of recipe videos on YouTube you can watch and rewatch over and over again. There are also countless cookery shows and even cookery channels on TV. Why is it that millions of people watch cooking shows every week yet hardly anyone actually tries to make the food? Come on – give it a try.

The bottom line is if you want to heal yourself then you need some basic cooking skills. If you want to beat the mad fat epidemic and regain your mind and your waistline then you need to start cooking, at least some of your food, from scratch. And I promise you it's much easier than you might think. Today we have Internet access to find recipes and watch how it's done and we have all the modern kitchen gadgets at our disposal. It doesn't need to be fancy, it just needs to have the right nutritious ingredients so you can ensure you are getting the right micronutrients to heal yourself once and for all.

Food for the Soul

I can honestly say I've come to love cooking. I love cooking for my son and our friends and family. It makes me feel happy. I know that every leaf of basil, clove of garlic, splash of apple cider vinegar, chopped onion and peeled carrot is feeding far more than our bellies. It is nourishing body, mind and spirit. The time spent and mindfulness of cooking is just another way of showing love. Cooking a meal is a sign of love to your partner, your family or to yourself. Good food really is the best medicine, and when we take the time to cook we nourish our body, mind and spirit.

Interestingly, cooking and baking classes are now being adopted by psychologists in the US for treating depressed and anxious patients. And a study published in the *British Journal of Occupational Therapy* in 2004 found that baking classes boosted confidence, increased concentration, and provided a sense of achievement for patients being treated in mental health clinics.

Cooking is a great way of boosting positive activity and it's personally rewarding when we see other people enjoying our food. It takes our mind off our problems and is a big step forward in the healing process. Once you understand the health benefits of the ingredients you use, it's almost as if you are making a pot of medicine rather than a pot of soup – a tonic or special potion you know is going to help heal your mind and lose weight.

> **Easy Step:** If you find yourself falling back into the trap of convenience foods reread chapter 6 to remind you of just how harmful processed foods are – and why they are making you mad and fat.

Music

Music is a sure-fire, fast-track mood changer for just about everyone. A certain song can take you back 20 years in the blink of an eye. A sad song can make you cry, a happy song can make you glad to be alive. Music affects us in a myriad of ways, far more than we could ever imagine. It helps us work through our problems, inspires creativity, affects our breathing, can reduce blood pressure, pain and alleviate stress. A study published in the *British Journal of Psychiatry* in 2011 showed that listening to music was cathartic and reduced symptoms of depression. Another study published in *JAMA Pediatrics* in 2013 found that music can help soothe emergency-room patients.

Music is sound and sound is rooted in vibration. Various vibroacoustic studies have been conducted over the years which show that music not only reduces depression but can ease the symptoms of Parkinson's disease and other debilitating disorders. Dr Lee Bartel, a music professor at the University of Toronto, is working with scientists around the world on new music therapy techniques to treat depression, fibromyalgia, Parkinson's and Alzheimer's and he says, 'Since the rhythmic pulses of music can drive and stabilise disorientation, we believe that low-frequency sound can help with these conditions.'

Studies show music can also help us to lose weight! Not only by motivating us to get more active but music can also distract us from what we might otherwise consider to be unpleasant – like going for a run, going to the gym or even for a walk. A study conducted at the Fairleigh Dickinson University's School of Psychology showed that women who walked while listening to music lost an average of 16 pounds, whereas those who did not listen to music while they walked only lost 8 pounds.

Have you ever wondered why you tend to drive faster when listening to a song you love? Or why you want to get up and dance when your favourite song comes on? This is because music releases dopamine in the brain (a mood-enhancing chemical) and studies show it increases by 9 per cent when we listen to music we enjoy. So get the tunes on! It doesn't matter if it's Lady Gaga, The Rolling Stones or Justin Bieber; so long as you enjoy what you are listening to then the music will elevate your mood and encourage you to be more active.

> *Easy Step:* Try adding music to your housework routine and sing and dance around your home – you'll feel better and get your house cleaned quicker!

> *Easy Step:* Singing is also great for mental health as it boosts the release of endorphins and oxytocin. So sing in the shower, in the car, or into a mirror holding a hairbrush – come on – admit it… we've all done it!

Essential oils

Instead of using scented candles, fragranced plug-ins and chemical diffusers, switch to burning essential oils. Many natural oils have proven healing properties, helping us to relax, detox, improve our mental health and even lose weight!

Johns Hopkins University in Baltimore and the Hebrew University of Jerusalem conducted a study into the healing power of frankincense and why it has psychoactive effects on the brain. Frankincense has been used since ancient times in religious ceremonies and as a powerful medicine – from Egyptian pharaohs to the three wise men in the Christian Nativity. The researchers discovered that incensole acetate – a resin from the plant that produces frankincense – influences the areas of the brain which regulate emotions. It activates the TRPV3 protein, a gene in human and animal brains which has an antidepressant and anti-anxiety effect. It effectively calms the brain and makes us feel more relaxed. Another great essential oil for mental health is rosemary. In fact, as mentioned before, studies show that smelling rosemary can increase memory by up to 75 per cent.

Peppermint oil relieves symptoms of depression and anxiety and can even help with weight loss. Dr Hirsch, a neurologist at the Smell and Taste Foundation in Chicago, conducted an experiment with 3,193 overweight volunteers. Each was given an inhaler containing scents and was asked to inhale three times into each nostril when they felt hungry. During the six-month study they didn't diet and ate two to four regular meals per day. On average they lost nearly five pounds per month – some people lost much more. Dr Hirsch reported, 'Some people lost so much weight we had to drop them from the programme.' The most effective scent used in the inhaler was peppermint oil.

> **Easy Step:** Invest in an inexpensive essential oil kit and burn oils to help you relax, think clearly and control hunger pangs as you make changes to your behaviour and diet.

Good vibrations

I hate going to the gym. Running on a treadmill is boring and working up a sweat in an oversized T-shirt surrounded by skinny girls in Lycra makes me feel more like Bridget Jones than Kelly Holmes. Even at school, I was the kid hiding behind the hill waiting to join the group on their last lap of the cross-country course. But even if you are like me and often try to avoid exercise, there is just no denying how good it is for us and recent studies show it is particularly good for our mental health.

Exercise is a powerful way to combat feelings of stress because it increases the level of key neurotransmitters like serotonin, dopamine and endorphins that often get depleted by anxiety, depression and a crap diet. That's why short bouts of exercise can boost our mood immediately – combating the negative feelings we experience when we're mad, fat or both. Neuroscientists have also discovered that exercise improves memory by encouraging the long-term growth of cells in the hippocampus – the part of our brains critical for long-term memory.

But what do we do if we hate exercising, don't have the cash for a health club membership, are too body conscious to go swimming and can't play tennis to save our life? We vibrate! No, I'm not talking about the battery-operated devices sold in adult sex shops; I'm talking about vibration plates, sometimes called 'power plates'. As the name would suggest, the vibration plate tones and defines muscle faster by using vibration rather than personal effort (always nice).

Research shows that vibration plates aid with weight loss and trim abdominal fat – harmful visceral fat between the organs. A study of obese women was conducted at the University of Antwerp in Belgium over a 12-month period. The women were split into four groups:

- Group 1 reduced their calorie intake but took no exercise.
- Group 2 reduced calories and took a conventional gym and fitness regime.
- Group 3 got the diet intervention plus vibration plate sessions lasting 15 minutes.
- Group 4 did not change their diet and took no exercise (the control group).

Over the year only the conventional fitness and vibration plate groups managed to lose weight and keep it off for the full year. The vibration group lost far more visceral fat than all the other groups, despite sessions only lasting for a maximum of 15 minutes. Another study at Holos University in Kansas showed that vibration plates reduced symptoms of depression and raised DHEA levels – a hormone produced in the adrenal gland which decreases with ageing. Low levels have been linked to depression, increased risk of cancer and many other degenerative disorders. The study showed that vibration plate therapy had a positive effect on the production of hormones and neurotransmitters and the massaging effect of vibration initiates an increase in dopamine and serotonin levels.

Vibration plates are inexpensive to buy, or can be hired on a weekly basis for less than the price of a bottle of wine. Unlike bulky treadmills and exercise bikes, they are relatively small, discreet, easy to use and you don't need to be on them for a long time to gain the benefit. Fifteen minutes is enough and they work! Plus vibration plates seem to be particularly effective at getting rid of visceral fat which has been linked to a whole host of health problems including metabolic disturbances, increased risk of cardiovascular disease, Type 2 diabetes and breast cancer. You can even vibrate while watching your favourite TV show.

Easy Step: Whatever you decide to do you need to move your body. Invest in a second-hand vibration plate, rent one to try it out, or simply get up and go for a short walk. If you currently do nothing, then start with a gentle few minutes and work your way up from there. Even a tiny amount of exercise, such as five to ten minutes, can make a huge difference to the way you look and feel.

Reiki

Reiki is a Japanese, energy-healing practice which is becoming very popular, even beyond the New Age community and hippie types. In fact, it is now being used in hospitals, hospices and medical centres to provide relief from numerous healthcare challenges including mental illness.

I first experienced reiki when I visited India many years ago – although in India it's known as pranic healing. I had visited a spa hoping a massage would ease my menstrual cramps but the girl performed pranic healing instead. I wasn't exactly sure what was happening when the girl lay me down and hovered her hands over my body but, despite her never touching me, I felt sensations in my legs and a warm feeling (as if I had a hot-water bottle attached to my belly). Amazingly, I felt really good after the treatment and was well enough to continue with our planned sightseeing excursions for the day. When I returned home I looked into this form of energy healing and it seems it has been used in medical practice since ancient times.

I discovered reference to 'laying on of hands' 24 times in the Bible. This type of intervention was used as medicine in ancient Egypt, Greece and China. There is even evidence from cave drawings that this type of healing was used in the Stone Age. Suffice to say this treatment has been around for a long time, and it certainly worked on me. I was so impressed by the results that I tried to find a teacher in Scotland – no easy task, as this was well before it became popular.

Eventually I found a lady who agreed to teach me, so I went on a course to learn how to do it. She had been taught reiki by a guy called William Lee Rand, the founder of The International Center for Reiki Training, and was one of the first people to bring reiki to the UK. To be honest, I found some of what she said a bit 'out there' and initially I thought she'd been having a wee puff of something before I had arrived! However, this woman really knew her stuff and what she taught me was invaluable and I have been using the technique to reduce stress and boost my energy levels ever since.

Another great thing about reiki is that you don't need to go to a fancy spa or salon and pay someone else – you can actually treat yourself by laying hands over different parts of your body. I know it sounds bonkers, but there's a whole bunch of studies on reiki which shows it really does work – especially for relief of anxiety, depression and stress.

Reiki means universal (rei) energy (ki), a form of vibrating energy – and while it may be more subtle than using the vibration plate or listening to music, it has a similar effect on our physical and mental health. Like the diet and nutrition, reiki has literally changed my life – it is safe and easy to learn, so why not give it a try?

Easy Step: You'd be amazed what you can find on YouTube…search for 'Learn reiki' and check out some of the free video tutorials for self-treatment. Alternatively, find a practitioner in your local area and schedule a session.

Mindfulness and meditation

For anyone who has seen the movie *Eat Pray Love,* based on Elizabeth Gilbert's book of the same name, you may remember Julia Roberts's struggle to meditate when her character visited an ashram in India. It's tricky to master and takes some getting used to. When I first tried meditation the chatter inside my brain just wouldn't stop. 'Have I done this, oh I forgot to do that, I must remember to pick up my dry cleaning, I've got a hole in my sock.' Seriously, you'd be amazed at the amount of nonsense that goes through your head every second of every minute of every day and you only notice it when you stop and try to meditate.

Sitting still and doing nothing while trying to empty your mind and not fall asleep is challenging for most people, but studies show that managing just a few minutes of mindfulness each day boasts a whole host of health benefits including reducing anxiety, mental stress and even weight loss! There are literally thousands of studies showing how good meditation is for us, yet in the West so few of us take the time to do it.

A study conducted in Belgium involving 400 students who followed an in-class mindfulness programme reported reduced indications of depression, anxiety and stress up to six months after their mindfulness training had stopped. Another study conducted by researchers at Oxford University showed that meditation is as good as antidepressants for tackling depression. The study followed 492 severely depressed adults over two years – half of them received mindfulness training and the other half stayed on antidepressants. The study findings showed that 44 per cent of people practising meditation slipped back into major depression compared with 47 per cent of people taking antidepressants. A Harvard MRI study proved that meditation literally rebuilds the brain's grey matter in eight weeks.

The secret to meditation is focusing on the present. Most of the thoughts flying through our minds are about the future or the past – thinking about what we want to do or remembering things we've already done. The easiest way to stay in the now is to simply focus your attention on your breath. Become aware of your chest breathing in and breathing out. Finding a quiet spot is also a good idea – so no TV, mobile phone buzzing, or radio playing in the background. You don't have to sit in the lotus position either, although it is very good for your posture. I've been known to meditate in the car or anywhere else I grab a bit of peace and quiet.

Easy Step: As always, start small – just a minute or two then build it up as you get better at quietening your mind. When your mind starts to wander, acknowledge the thought and just let it go. I sometimes picture the thoughts floating out of my head in a bubble until they pop. It takes a bit of getting used to but people who regularly meditate report they are happier, healthier and their relationships are stronger. It costs nothing and only takes a few minutes of your time each day. And when you get really good at it you can meditate anywhere. If a butterfly brain like me can do it – anyone can!

Chapter 11: The Future – You Can Do It!

'Here's to the wild, the weird, and the wonderful . . .
To the rebels that were not born to fit in but to gloriously stand out . . .
Here's to the magical, the mystical, and the misunderstood . . .
To those who read the compass written on the walls of their hearts . . .
and follow the North star etched upon their spirit . . .
Here's to the wild ones. Here's to you . . .'

– C. Ara Campbell
Ode to Misfits

After reading this book you may be feeling a bit overwhelmed or shocked and I don't blame you. When it comes to good health and how to achieve it, we have often been misinformed or tricked into believing certain foods are good for us when scientific evidence now reveals this just isn't true. In some cases, the new information simply hasn't filtered out to the people who so desperately need it. Instead it remains effectively hidden in academic or scientific documents that are largely incomprehensible to anyone without a PhD. In other cases, this lack of new, more relevant information has been suppressed or dismissed by vested interests keen to maintain the status quo and excessive profits – often at the expense of our physical and mental health.

We have also been let down by our governments who have failed to provide doctors with accurate information about the medicines they prescribe – including transparent access to *all* the clinical trial data around those medications. Governments have also systematically failed to tackle the inappropriate power and influence exercised by 'big food' and 'big pharma' on government policy.

But as the old saying goes, 'You can't make the same mistake twice. The second time you make it, it's not a mistake, it's a choice.' So with this in mind . . .

Forget what you've been told as fact. We need to stop listening to experts and assuming everything they say is 100 per cent correct – even when they have letters after their name and wear a white coat. And that goes for this book too. Don't just accept what I am saying is fact either – investigate it for yourself. Go online – we have access to more scientific research now than at any point in human history. Start trusting yourself and your own body. Be a rebel – gloriously stand out and take your health back once and for all.

I've been where you may be right now – whether you are currently struggling with your weight, mental health or both. I remember a time when just getting through the day was all I could manage; I remember wondering, 'Is this it? Is this seriously the best I can hope for?' It can be exhausting and demoralising and I would often reach for foods to comfort me through my pain. It took me years to realise that even the so-called healthy food I was eating was contributing to my pain!

I hope this book has made you angry – *really* angry. I also hope you are excited, filled with optimism and inspired to regain your mental and physical health.

If you are overweight, chances are you have tried numerous diets and your failure to make any lasting change just amplified your apathy and distress. If you're currently overweight – it's not your fault. You've been fighting the wrong battles based on calories and fat content instead of micronutrients and good quality. Just shift your focus and experience the results for yourself.

If you are currently on antidepressants you may have been too scared to come off these addictive drugs. Besides, the blandness of life on the drugs is better than the hell off them – right? But it doesn't have to be this way. Again, shift your focus to micronutrients and food quality – when you do you will start to feel and look better. And when you start to feel better you will find the strength to wean yourself off the drugs once and for all.

I know it's possible – I did it, and if I can so can you.

This book is about so much more than just our individual health.

It is a call to action.

It is a rallying cry for all of us to be better parents, better partners and better people – to become conscious again. We simply must stop sleepwalking through our day, especially in terms of what we buy and what we eat.

We need to educate ourselves and our loved ones. We need to pull back the façade of big business and expensive, slick marketing and see the food we eat through new eyes and question exactly what it is we are putting in our shopping trolleys. Next time you go food shopping ask yourself – what drew me to the product? Why did I pick it up? What's in the product? How many ingredients does it have? How many can I pronounce? We need to wake up, take responsibility and understand the connection between what we eat, how we feel, how we look and what's going on in the world as a result of our purchase.

Of course we all need our little treats and I'm certainly not going to stop enjoying my glass of wine or dark chocolate ginger biscuits! But for mealtime grocery shopping we must start looking beyond the label and trusting the facts and our own intuition as to what is good for us and what is making us mad and fat. Hopefully the information I've shared in this book will help.

We also need to start thinking in terms of balance. My granddad smoked cigarettes and drank whisky but my granny's nutrient-rich cooking, the daily preventative medicine routine, and a steady supply of fresh vegetables from the allotment ensured his diet was jam-packed with micronutrients which helped to mitigate the negative effect of his unhealthy habits. If we've enjoyed the Friday night 'blowout' of takeaway food, chocolate cake and a bucketload of wine, it makes sense to move more on Saturday to shake off the cobwebs of a hangover and burn off a few of those excess calories. It also makes sense to consider topping up on the micronutrients that were missing from Friday's choices to ensure we counteract any 'Big 4' deficiencies or inflammation caused by our splurge. Remember the car analogy from chapter 6 and get into the habit of monitoring your micronutrient intake and not just the amount of fat, calories and carbohydrates you consume. In an ideal world retailers and food manufacturers would state the amount of vitamins, minerals and essential fatty acids on the nutrition guidelines of packaging but they won't do this unless our governments force them to. That's extremely unlikely because big food corporations don't want to tell you how nutritionally devoid their products really are and unfortunately our politicians are often ineffective given the power big business has over them. So, we need to do this for ourselves.

Time and time again Western governments have dished out bad dietary advice, often steered by big food or pharmaceutical companies looking to boost profits. Even today, Britain's health authorities are considering whether to allow processed foods to carry the official 5-a-day logo, an emblem which is currently restricted to foods which are 100 per cent fruit or vegetable. So many shoppers and busy mums rely on the five-a-day logo to guide them on buying healthy products and our kids are also taught about the benefits of five-a-day in school. Adding this logo to processed food makes no sense and is misleading to consumers. Most processed food contains ingredients that usually have not been living for months, and those often inferior ingredients are then pulverised, modified, cooked at high temperatures during manufacture and mixed with a whole bunch of additives, preservatives and other chemicals. The end result is a product stripped of what little micronutrients were present at the start of production and completely unrecognisable to the fruits and vegetables we would expect behind the 'healthy' five-a-day message. Oh, and guess who is sitting on the 'external reference group' advising the Department of Health on the change to five-a-day criteria? Yep, you guessed it – representatives from food processing manufacturers and non-government organisations sponsored by 'big food'. Once again, the British government is on the cusp of making yet another food policy decision based on guidance coming from corporations trying to either 'game the system' or processed food manufacturers with a financial interest in regulatory change.

This bad advice has left so many of us struggling under the weight of the mad fat epidemic with pharmaceutical companies all too ready to step in with their products to manage our symptoms. America now has the highest obesity rate in the world and it's also number one for prescription drug use. A study conducted by the famous Mayo Clinic found that 7 out of every 10 Americans took at least one prescription drug – that's 70 per cent of the population! More than half of the population take two prescription medications, and 20 per cent are on at least five prescription medications! And Britain isn't far behind, with almost 50 per cent of Brits taking prescription drugs. This is far from normal and an unacceptable statistic for countries listed as among the wealthiest in the world.

In economic terms, we may be rich and powerful but when it comes to our health the West often ranks lower than developing nations. In parts of Glasgow where I live the life expectancy is now lower than some Third World countries; in fact, the World Health Organization has even created a term for this health problem, calling it 'The Glasgow Effect'. Cigarettes and alcohol play a big part in 'The Glasgow Effect' but diet has also been identified as a driving factor, with poverty cited as the main overarching cause. The average life expectancy for a man living in the east end of Glasgow is now just 63, far less than the 'three score and ten' most of us expect as a bare minimum, and 20 years short of my grandparents' lifespan. And although it is easy to point the finger at poverty – deprivation has been an issue in Glasgow for generations and it didn't stop my grandparents from living to a ripe old age. Just like Americans, twenty-first-century Glaswegians no longer consume enough micronutrients in their food and this is why so many of us are sick, fat and taking antidepressants to manage the symptoms of our dwindling mental health.

American author, food writer and professor at UC Berkeley Michael Pollan famously wrote in one of his books 'Better to pay the grocer than the doctor' and this makes perfect sense. If we don't get enough vitamins, minerals, amino acids, protein and omega-3 fatty acids in our diet then it is only a matter a time before we get sick and need to visit the doctor. But the good news is we don't have to pay more to eat well if we get educated and understand the *true* quality of food we consume. Poverty is always rolled out as an excuse for folk eating a poor diet, but unless you are living in a famine-stricken country in Africa it absolutely doesn't have to be the case. My grandparents got by on a shoestring budget yet ate wholesome, nutrient-rich food every day. And as evidenced by the experiment with my friend – cooking from scratch with good-quality ingredients can actually save you money.

We may believe that it's more expensive to buy better-quality, traditionally produced or organic food, but most Brits and Americans waste around 40 per cent of the food we buy anyway. A little meal planning could easily cancel out any additional cost. And even if you are strapped for cash at the end of the month before payday, a pot of hearty home-made soup and crusty bread is more cost effective and far better for you than picking up packets of 'low-fat' noodles, pasta mixes or other heavily processed food as a cheap meal solution. Instinctively we all know this – right? Most of us do understand what is good for us yet so often we continue to make the same mistakes because we fall for the clever marketing in supermarkets and bad advice from our governments. I certainly did until I realised the impact it was having on my waistline and mental health.

The relationship between 'big food' and 'big pharma' is a marriage made in hell and our governments are fanning the flames with their laissez-faire approach to food and medicine. This toxic triangle is a dance between directors of food and drug companies working hard to serve their shareholders, and politicians being steered by corporations or, worse, are in their back pocket.

We have put our trust in a system which is geared towards profit growth rather than safeguarding the health of Western nations. And the result is the mad fat epidemic. Our increased reliance on antidepressants and antibiotics to cope with the fallout from 'big food' is further compounding the problem by lining the pockets of 'big pharma' – creating an endless cycle of despair for millions of Western women. And of course these medications are dumbing us down, making it all the more difficult for us to lose weight and think straight so we can finally put an end to this madness! The only way we can escape is to take back control of our own health by providing our body and brain with the vital nutrients they need to function properly. It really is down to us to heal ourselves – nobody else is going to do it for us.

Your time is now – right now. The past is the past, today is a new day and you can change your future by reclaiming your power as the wild and wonderful woman you are. You *can* heal yourself and help to reverse the tide of ill health by eating the 'right food', supporting the 'good guys' growing food in your community, and by using your purse power to demand better-quality, safe and nutritious food from supermarkets. What we all must realise is that we drive the market by the choices we make when buying food. If we stop buying crap food then it will no longer be profitable for 'big food' to make it and they will be forced to change their ways. While it may appear we are powerless to effect change nothing could be further from the truth. 'Big food' needs our money to drive their profits, and once we stop handing over our hard-earned cash they will soon get the message and adapt accordingly. We are already seeing signs of this in the US with some of the big meat processors committing to using less antibiotics in livestock production and McDonald's in Canada promising to sell 'sustainable beef'. These guys didn't wake up one morning and suddenly develop a conscience. They were driven to change because consumers demanded that change. We control the market by the choices we make and we must never lose sight of that.

Women hold a huge amount of influence. We influence our children and we usually decide what our family eats. Most of us do the weekly grocery shopping and the majority of the cooking so we hold the key to health and well-being – not just for us, but for our family too. We all have an important role in this world but we need to step up and take responsibility. If we just take the time to get educated and become mindful of what we eat, how we live and what we buy, we won't just be able to regain our health but seize new opportunities that could radically improve our lives.

Remember; keep your eye on the prize – a healthy body and a sane mind. Use that goal to drive you forward. Start to visualise all the things you may be able to achieve once you feel better. See it clearly in your mind's eye. Some of us might imagine having a hot bikini body so we can strip off during summer without always reaching for the beach towel to cover up our lumps and bumps. That's fine if you use it as a positive incentive. But what about the real life-enhancing things you could do once you have more get-up-and-go and can think clearly? Maybe take that evening class you previously didn't have the energy for. Go for a promotion at work – employers are more likely to hire someone who looks great, feels great and thinks straight. Or get a new, better job – especially if your boss is part of the 'clutter' we discussed in chapter 10. Even the simple things like spending *real* quality time with your friends and family – connecting with them in a more meaningful way instead of being wrapped up in your own head, immersed in your own problems. How would your relationships change if you finally had the capacity to really be there for your loved ones? Think of the self-respect you will feel for knowing that you healed yourself, not someone in a white coat ushering you out the door with another prescription. Consider how proud you will feel when *you* become the role model who inspires others to heal themselves too, when people respond more positively to the 'new you' – or the 'old you' that just got lost for a while.

At the 2009 peace conference in Vancouver the Dalai Lama

announced 'The world will be saved by the Western woman' and I couldn't agree more. His comment and this book are a call to action to all of us girls in the West. In the West we often have more freedom and greater equality than many women in other parts of the world. So let's use our freedom to reverse the tide of ill health sweeping across Western nations and put an end to the damage being caused by 'big food' and 'big pharma'.

Just as our grannies kept the home fires burning during two world wars and the Great Depression, let's join hands across the Atlantic and beyond and embrace the call to action together. Let's stand up as the powerful women we are, take back control of our minds and bodies, and kick this mad fat epidemic into touch. And once we do that for ourselves, let's share our knowledge and wisdom with others, just as our grannies passed their insights down to us. We really are what we eat. If we change what we eat we can change ourselves. And if we do that we might just change the world!

References

This section contains all the references and scientific evidence and research papers to back up what I've said in the book, including online links where possible. The links will take you to the full paper or abstracts; some must be purchased but they will provide a great starting place if you want to investigate further. To minimise space if there were more than three authors in the paper I've used the lead author followed by 'et al.' to indicate more people were involved in the research. This material is deliberately at the back, rather than in the text, because often references can interrupt the flow of the book and make it look a bit academic and intimidating. I want this book to be simple and easy to follow, but also backed up by science should you want to investigate further – indeed, what's listed here is just a snapshot of what exists online. So dive in and investigate for yourself. All websites were checked for accuracy 28/1/2016.

Introduction: Reality Check

1. Allen V., Awford J. (2014) Girl, 4, went into anaphylactic shock and lost consciousness on a plane after selfish passenger ignored three warnings not to eat nuts on board. *Daily Mail* http://www.dailymail.co.uk/news/article-2724684/Nut-allergy-girl-went-anaphylactic-shock-plane-passenger-ignored-three-warnings-not-eat-nuts-board.html
2. Allergy Statistics from Allergy UK website https://www.allergyuk.org/allergy-statistics/allergy-statistics
3. Allergy Statistics and Facts from WebMed website http://www.webmd.com/allergies/allergy-statistics
4. Attention Deficit Hyperactivity Disorder (ADHD) from Centers for Disease Control and Prevention (CDC) website http://www.cdc.gov/nchs/fastats/adhd.htm
5. Mental Health Statistics from Young Minds website http://www.youngminds.org.uk/training_services/policy/mental_health_statistics
6. Milmo C. (2015) 'Dietary advice from the 1970s found to be a big fat mistake.' *Independent* http://www.independent.co.uk/life-style/health-

and-families/health-news/dietary-advice-from-the-1970s-found-to-be-a-big-fat-mistake-10034786.html

7. Spencer B. (2015) 'Low-fat diets do NOT work: Scientists cast doubt on years of health advice after concluding there is no evidence that reducing fat intake helps cut weight'. *Daily Mail* http://www.dailymail.co.uk/health/article-3296075/Trying-lose-weight-Ditch-low-fat-diet-Scientists-cast-doubt-years-health-advice-concluding-no-evidence-reducing-fat-intake-helps-cut-weight.html

Chapter 1: Mad Fat Epidemic

1. Bindley K. (2011) 'women and prescription drugs: one in four takes mental health meds'. *Huffington Post* http://www.huffingtonpost.com/2011/11/16/women-and-prescription-drug-use_n_1098023.html

2. Bekiempis V. (2011) 'Why one in four women is on psych meds.' *The Guardian* http://www.theguardian.com/commentisfree/cifamerica/2011/nov/21/one-in-four-women-psych-meds

3. Mental Health Statistics Young Minds Website http://www.youngminds.org.uk/training_services/policy/mental_health_statistics

4. Berthoud R. (2011) 'Trends in the employment of disabled people in Britain.' Institute of Social and Economic Research https://www.iser.essex.ac.uk/files/iser_working_papers/2011-03.pdf

5. Compassion in World Farming website (2013) 'The Life of: Broiler Chickens https://www.ciwf.org.uk/media/5235306/The-life-of-Broiler-chickens.pdf

6. Bell D. D., Weaver W. D. eds (2002) *Commercial Chicken Meat and Egg Production.* New York: Springer 5th edition

7. Quart M. D. et al. (1992) 'Effects of poultry fat and yellow grease on broiler performance and profitability'. 'Poultry Science. v71(5): 821–828 http://ps.oxfordjournals.org/content/71/5/821.abstract?related-urls=yes&legid=poultrysci;71/5/821&cited-by=yes&legid=poultrysci;71/5/821

8. BBC News (2006) 'Mental Health Link to Diet Change' http://news.bbc.co.uk/1/hi/health/4610070.stm

9. Cornah D. 'The Mental Health Foundation Feeding Minds: The Impact of Food on Mental Health' https://www.mentalhealth.org.uk/sites/default/files/Feeding-Minds.pdf

10. Simopoulos A. P. (2002) 'The importance of the ratio of omega-6/omega-3 essential fatty acids.' *Biomed Pharmacother.* Oct v56(8):365–79 http://www.ncbi.nlm.nih.gov/pubmed/12442909

11. Chalmers A. G., Sinclair A. H., Carver M. (1998) *HGCA Cereals Research Review.* No. 41: Nutrients other than NPK for cereals: A review

12. http://cereals.ahdb.org.uk/media/411719/rr41_complete_final_report.pdf

13. Fan M. S. et al. (2008) 'Evidence of decreasing mineral density in wheat grain over the last 160 years.' *J Trace Elem Med Biol.* v22(4):315–24 http://www.ncbi.nlm.nih.gov/pubmed/19013359

14. Ensminger M. E., Ensminger A. H. (1993) *Foods & Nutrition Encyclopedia*, Two Volume Set. CRC Press 2nd edition

15. Beyreuther K. et al. (2007) 'Consensus meeting: monosodium glutamate – an update.' *Eur J Clin Nutr.* v61:304–13. http://www.nature.com/ejcn/journal/v61/n3/abs/1602526a.html

16. Afifi M. M., Abbas A. M. (2011) 'Monosodium glutamate versus diet induced obesity in pregnant rats and their offspring.' *Acta Physiol Hung.* Jun v98(2):177–88. http://www.ncbi.nlm.nih.gov/pubmed/21616776

17. Bachmanov A. A. et al. (2009) 'Glutamate taste and appetite in laboratory mice: physiologic and genetic analyses.' *Am J Clin Nutr.* Sep v90(3):756S–763S. http://www.ncbi.nlm.nih.gov/pubmed/19571213

18. Bunyan J., Murrell E. A., Shah P. P. (1976) 'The induction of obesity in rodents by means of monosodium glutamate.' *Br J Nutr.* Jan v35(1):25–39. http://www.ncbi.nlm.nih.gov/pubmed/1106764

19. Collison K. S. et al. (2009) 'Effect of dietary monosodium glutamate on trans fat-induced nonalcoholic fatty liver disease.' *J Lipid Res.* Aug v50(8):1521–37. http://www.ncbi.nlm.nih.gov/pubmed/19001666

20. Collison K. S. et al. (2012) 'Nutrigenomics of hepatic steatosis in a feline model: effect of monosodium glutamate, fructose, and trans-fat feeding.' *Genes Nutr.* Apr v7(2):265–80. http://www.ncbi.nlm.nih.gov/pubmed/22144172

21. Farombi E. O., Onyema O. O. (2006) 'Monosodium glutamate-induced oxidative damage and genotoxicity in the rat: modulatory role of vitamin C, vitamin E and quercetin.' *Hum Exp Toxicol.* May v25(5):251–9. http://www.ncbi.nlm.nih.gov/pubmed/16758767

22. Freeman M. (2006) 'Reconsidering the effects of monosodium glutamate: a literature review.' *J Am Acad Nurse Pract.* Oct v18(10):482–6. http://www.ncbi.nlm.nih.gov/pubmed/16999713

23. Geha R. S. et al. (2000) 'Review of alleged reaction to monosodium glutamate and outcome of a multicenter double-blind placebo-controlled study.' *J Nutr.* Apr v130(4S Suppl):1058S-62S. http://www.ncbi.nlm.nih.gov/pubmed/10736382

24. Hermanussen M. et al. (2006) 'Obesity, voracity, and short stature: the impact of glutamate on the regulation of appetite.' *Eur J Clin Nutr.* Jan v60(1):25–31. http://www.nature.com/ejcn/journal/v60/n1/full/1602263a.html?message=remove

25. Insawang T. et al. (2012) 'Monosodium glutamate (MSG) intake is associated with the prevalence of metabolic syndrome in a rural Thai population.' *Nutr Metab.* Jun v9(1):50 http://www.ncbi.nlm.nih.gov/

pubmed/22681873

26. Iwase M. et al. (2000) 'Effects of monosodium glutamate-induced obesity in spontaneously hypertensive rats vs. Wistar Kyoto rats: serum leptin and blood flow to brown adipose tissue.' *Hypertens Res.* Sep v23(5):503–10. http://medicalcorps.org/rat-1.htm

27. Kondoh T., Torii K. (2008) 'MSG intake suppresses weight gain, fat deposition, and plasma leptin levels in male Sprague-Dawley rats.' *Physiol Behav.* Sep v95(1-2):135–44. https://www.researchgate.net/publication/5296014_MSG_intake_suppresses_weight_gain_fat_deposition_and_plasma_leptin_levels_in_male_Sprague-Dawley_rats

28. Kondoh T., Tsurugizawa T., Torii K. (2009) 'Brain functional changes in rats administered with monosodium L-glutamate in the stomach.' *Ann N Y Acad Sci.* Jul v1170:77–81. http://onlinelibrary.wiley.com/doi/10.1111/j.1749-6632.2009.03884.x/abstract

29. Kondoh T., Mallick H. N., Torii K. (2009) 'Activation of the gut-brain axis by dietary glutamate and physiologic significance in energy homeostasis.' *Am J Clin Nutr.* Sep v90(3):832S–7S.

30. http://www.ncbi.nlm.nih.gov/pubmed/19587084

31. Loliger J. (2000) 'Function and importance of glutamate for savory foods.' *J Nutr.* Apr v130(4S Suppl):915S–20S. http://intl-jn.nutrition.org/content/130/4/915S.full

32. Otsubo H. et al. (2011) 'Induction of Fos expression in the rat forebrain after intragastric administration of monosodium L-glutamate, glucose and NaCl.' *Neuroscience.* Nov v196:97–103. https://www.researchgate.net/publication/51654480_Induction_of_Fos_expression_in_the_rat_forebrain_after_intragastric_administration_of_monosodium_L-glutamate_glucose_and_NaCl

33. Simopoulos A. P. (2006). 'Evolutionary aspects of diet, the omega-6/omega-3 ratio and genetic variation: nutritional implications for chronic diseases.' *Biomedicine & Pharmacology.* v60(9):502–7 http://www.sciencedirect.com/science/article/pii/S0753332206002435

34. Witting L. A., Lee L. (1975) 'Recommended dietary allowance for vitamin E: relation to dietary, erythrocyte and adipose tissue linoleate.' *Am J Clin Nutr.* Jun v28(6):577–83 http://www.ncbi.nlm.nih.gov/pubmed/1130317

35. Ren J. et al. (2008) 'Composition of adipose tissue and marrow fat in humans by ^{1}H NMR at 7 Tesla.' *J Lipid Res.* v49(9):2055–62 http://www.ncbi.nlm.nih.gov/pmc/articles/PMC2515528/

36. London S. J. et al. (1991) 'Fatty acid composition of subcutaneous adipose tissue and diet in postmenopausal US women.' *Am J Clin Nutr.* Aug v53(2):340–5 http://www.ncbi.nlm.nih.gov/pubmed/1858698

37. Garland M. et al. (1998) 'The relation between dietary intake and adipose tissue composition of selected fatty acids in US women.' *Am J Clin Nutr.* Jan v67(1):25–30 http://www.ncbi.nlm.nih.gov/pubmed/9440371

38. Berry E. M. et al. (1986) 'The relationship of dietary fat to plasma lipid levels as studied by factor analysis of adipose tissue fatty acid composition in a free-living population of middle-aged American men.' *Am J Clin Nutr.* Aug v44(2):220–31 http://www.ncbi.nlm.nih.gov/pubmed/3728359

39. Knutsen S. F. et al. (2003) 'Comparison of adipose tissue fatty acids with dietary fatty acids as measured by 24-hour recall and food frequency questionnaire in Black and White Adventists: the Adventist Health Study.' *Ann Epidemiol.* Feb v13(2):119–27 http://www.ncbi.nlm.nih.gov/pubmed/12559671

40. Aihaud G. et al. (2006) 'Temporal changes in dietary fats: role of n-6 polyunsaturated fatty acids in excessive adipose tissue development and relationship to obesity.' *Progress in Lipid Research.* May v45(3):203–36 http://www.sciencedirect.com/science/article/pii/S016378270600004X

41. Onyema O. O. et al. (2006) 'Effect of vitamin E on monosodium glutamate induced hepatotoxicity and oxidative stress in rats.' *Indian J Biochem Biophys.* Feb v43(1):20–4. http://www.ncbi.nlm.nih.gov/pubmed/16955747

42. Pavlovic V., Sarac M. (2010) 'The role of ascorbic acid and monosodium glutamate in thymocyte apoptosis.' *Bratisl Lek Listy.* v111(6):357–60. http://www.ncbi.nlm.nih.gov/pubmed/20635684

43. Platt S. R. (2007) 'The role of glutamate in central nervous system health and disease–a review.' *Vet J.* Mar v173(2):278–86. http://www.ncbi.nlm.nih.gov/pubmed/16376594

44. Ren X. et al. (2011) 'Effects of ad libitum ingestion of monosodium glutamate on weight gain in C57BL6/J mice.' *Digestion.* v83(Suppl 1):32–6. http://www.ncbi.nlm.nih.gov/pubmed/21389726

45. Smriga M. (2007) 'COFAG comments on: "Monosodium glutamate-induced oxidative damage and genotoxicity in the rat: modulatory role of vitamin C, vitamin E and quercetin".' *Hum Exp Toxicol.* Oct v26(10):833–4; author reply 835-6. http://www.ncbi.nlm.nih.gov/pubmed/18025056

46. Tarasoff L., Kelly M. F. (1993) 'Monosodium L-glutamate: a double-blind study and review.' *Food Chem Toxicol.* Dec v31(12):1019–35. http://www.ncbi.nlm.nih.gov/pubmed/8282275

47. Walker R., Lupien J. R. (2000) 'The safety evaluation of monosodium glutamate.' *J Nutr.* Apr v130(4S Suppl):1049S–52S. http://intl-jn.nutrition.org/content/130/4/1049S.full

48. Yang D. et al. (2012) '*Lycium barbarum* extracts protect the brain from blood-brain barrier disruption and cerebral edema in experimental stroke.' *PLoS One.* v7(3):e33596. http://www.ncbi.nlm.nih.gov/pmc/articles/PMC3306421/

49. 'Corn Production in the United States' https://en.wikipedia.org/wiki/Corn_production_in_the_United_States

50. Harcombe Z. et al. (2015) 'Evidence from randomised controlled trials

did not support the introduction of dietary fat guidelines in 1977 and 1983: a systematic review and meta-analysis.' *Open Heart.* v2(1) http://openheart.bmj.com/content/2/1/e000196.abstract?sid=7217c2a8-513e-4e7e-837a-fe5389053fde

51. Tobias D. K. et al. (2015) 'Effect of low-fat diet interventions versus other diet interventions on long-term weight change in adults: a systematic review and meta-analysis' *Lancet Diabetes Endocrinol.* http://press.thelancet.com/diet.pdf

52. Wehrwein P. (2011) 'Astounding increase in antidepressant use by Americans.' *Harvard Health Blog* http://www.health.harvard.edu/blog/astounding-increase-in-antidepressant-use-by-americans-201110203624

53. A National Statistics Publication for Scotland (2014) 'Medicines for Mental Health' http://www.isdscotland.org/Health-Topics/Prescribing-and-Medicines/Publications/2014-09-30/2014-09-30-PrescribingMentalHealth-report.pdf

54. Stoller-Conrad J. (2015) 'Microbes help produce serotonin in gut.' *caltech* https://www.caltech.edu/news/microbes-help-produce-serotonin-gut-46495

55. Markets and Markets Press Release (2014) 'Global Market for Weight Loss Worth US$586.3 Billion by 2014.' http://www.marketsandmarkets.com/PressReleases/global-market-for-weight-loss-worth-$726-billion-by-2014.asp

56. World Health Organization (2009) *Calcium and Magnesium in Drinking Water: Public Health Significance.* Geneva: World Health Organization Press http://www.who.int/water_sanitation_health/publications/publication_9789241563550/en/

57. Forrest K. Y. and Stuhldreher W. L. (2011) 'Prevalence and correlates of vitamin D deficiency in US adults.' *Nutrition Research*, Jan v31(1):48–54. http://www.ncbi.nlm.nih.gov/pubmed/21310306

58. Pearce S. H. S. and Cheetham T. D. (2011) 'Diagnosis and management of vitamin D deficiency.' *BMJ Clinical Edition.* Jan v340:142–7. https://weblearn.ox.ac.uk/access/content/group/b6eb0442-7719-4f6f-b0da-f36b91c6c235/BM1%20Year%202%20Learning%20resources/Calcium%20regulation/Vit%20D%20review%20BMJ%20Pearce%202010.pdf

59. Alliance for Natural Health website (2009) 'Vitamin C Deficiency Worse than Feared: Research News' http://anhinternational.org/2009/09/10/vitamin-c-deficiency-worse-than-feared-research-news/

60. Leung W. C. et al. (2009) 'Two common single nucleotide polymorphisms in the gene encoding beta-carotene 15,15%u2019-monoxygenase alter beta-carotene metabolism in female volunteers.' *The FASEB Journal.* Apr v23(4):1041–53 http://www.ncbi.nlm.nih.gov/pubmed/19103647

Chapter 2: The War on Food

1. 'Economic History of the UK' https://en.wikipedia.org/wiki/Economic_history_of_the_United_Kingdom

2. Hayward R. A. et al. (2006) 'Narrative review: lack of evidence for recommended low-density lipoprotein treatment targets: a solvable problem.' *Annuls of Internal Medicine.* v145(7):520–30. http://annals.org/article.aspx?articleid=729152

3. Hodgekiss A., Spencer B. (2016) 'EXCLUSIVE: how big pharma greed is killing tens of thousands around the world: patients are over-medicated and often given profitable drugs with "little proven benefits", leading doctors warn.' *Daily Mail* http://www.dailymail.co.uk/health/article-3460321/How-Big-Pharma-greed-killing-tens-thousands-world-Patients-medicated-given-profitable-drugs-little-proven-benefits-leading-doctors-warn.html

4. Malnick E. et al. (2016) 'Ministers launch urgent inquiry into NHS officials' second jobs at drugs firms.' *Telegraph* http://www.telegraph.co.uk/news/nhs/12160260/NHS-officials-with-second-jobs-at-drug-firms.html

5. Malnick E. et al. (2016) 'Pharmaceutical firms paying members of panel which oversees NHS drug procurement.' *Telegraph* http://www.telegraph.co.uk/news/nhs/12162032/Third-of-panel-overseeing-NHS-drugs-procurement-being-paid-by-pharmaceutical-firms.html

6. Cameron D. (2010) Speech 'Rebuilding trust in politics' 8 February 2010

7. Represent.us website Study: 'Congress Literally Doesn't Care what you think.' https://represent.us/action/theproblem-4/

8. 'Latest Stats from Trussell Trust website' https://www.trusselltrust.org/news-and-blog/latest-stats/

9. Fernandez C. and Ellicott C. (2015) 'TV chef's war on the stores that demand the perfect parsnip.' *Daily Mail* http://www.dailymail.co.uk/news/article-3301223/TV-chef-s-war-stores-demand-perfect-parsnip.html

Chapter 3: A Brief History of Medicine

1. Meikle J. (2015) 'Doctors write 10m needless antibiotics prescriptions a year, says Nice'. *The Guardian* http://www.theguardian.com/society/2015/aug/18/soft-touch-doctors-write-10m-needless-prescriptions-a-year-says-nice

2. Blaser M. (2011) 'Antibiotic overuse: stop the killing of beneficial bacteria.' *Nature.* v476: 393–4 (25 August 2011) http://www.nature.com/nature/journal/v476/n7361/full/476393a.html

3. Asociación RUVID (2013) 'Effects of antibiotics on gut flora analyzed.' *ScienceDaily.* 9 January 2013 http://www.sciencedaily.com/releases/2013/01/130109081145.htm

4.	'Eat more yogurt! Low levels of healthy gut bacteria could be the cause of mental health issues such as "anxiety and schizophrenia"' (2015) *Daily Mail* http://www.dailymail.co.uk/news/article-2419418/Low-levels-healthy-gut-bacteria-cause-mental-health-issues-anxiety-schizophrenia-say-scientists.html

5.	Anderson R. (2014) 'Pharmaceutical industry gets high on fat profits.' *BBC News* http://www.bbc.co.uk/news/business-28212223

6.	Gøtzsche P. (2015) 'Prescription pills are Britain's third biggest killer: side-effects of drugs taken for insomnia and anxiety kill thousands. Why do doctors hand them out like Smarties?' *Daily Mail* http://www.dailymail.co.uk/health/article-3234334/Prescription-pills-Britain-s-biggest-killer-effects-drugs-taken-insomnia-anxiety-kill-thousands-doctors-hand-like-Smarties.html

7.	Murray, C. and Lopez, A. (1996) *The Global Burden of Disease: A Comprehensive Assessment of Mortality and Disability from Diseases, Injuries, and Risk Factors in 1990 and Projected to 2020: Summary* (Global burden of disease and injury series) Cambridge, Massachusetts: Harvard University Press

8.	World Federation for Mental Health report (2012) 'Health Depression: A Global Crisis' http://www.who.int/mental_health/management/depression/wfmh_paper_depression_wmhd_2012.pdf

9.	'What do doctors know about nutrition?' (1988) *Nutrition & Food Science*, Vol. v88(1)12–12 http://www.emeraldinsight.com/doi/abs/10.1108/eb059164?journalCode=nfs&

10.	Goldacre B. (2012) *Bad Pharma: How Drug Companies Mislead Doctors and Harm Patients*. London, Forth Estate

11.	Gultekin F. et al. (2013) 'The effects of food and food additives on behaviour.' *International Journal of Health and Nutrition*, v4(1):21–32 http://www.academia.edu/5312057/The_Effects_of_Food_and_Food_Additives_on_Behaviors_INTRODUCTION

12.	Hodgekiss A., Spencer B. (2016) 'EXCLUSIVE: how big pharma greed is killing tens of thousands around the world: patients are over-medicated and often given profitable drugs with "little proven benefits,"leading doctors warn.' *Daily Mail* http://www.dailymail.co.uk/health/article-3460321/How-Big-Pharma-greed-killing-tens-thousands-world-Patients-medicated-given-profitable-drugs-little-proven-benefits-leading-doctors-warn.html

Chapter 4: Time to Get Angry

1.	'The Century of the Self – Part 1 of 4 – Happiness Machine' (The story of Edward Bernays) (2015) http://www.dailymotion.com/video/x2j2sfp

2.	Wansink B. (2006) *Mindless Eating: Why We Eat More Than We Think*. New York: Bantam-Dell

3. Argo J. J., White K. (2012) When do consumers eat more? The role of appearance self-esteem and food packaging Cues.' *Journal of Marketing* Mar v 76(2): 67–80. 76 http://www.sauder.ubc.ca/Faculty/People/Faculty_ Members/~/media/9084A58B9D204A2CBC17E95C87990DF8.ashx

4. Barkeling B. et al. (2003) 'Vision and eating behavior in obese subjects.' *Obesity Research* v 11(1):130–4. http://onlinelibrary.wiley.com/ doi/10.1038/oby.2003.21/full

5. Baumeister R. F. (2002) 'Yielding to temptation: self-control failure, impulsive purchasing, and Consumer Behavior.' *Journal of Consumer Research*. Marv28(4):670–6http://www.jstor.org/stable/10.1086/338209

6. Baumeister R. F., Heatherton T. F. (1996) 'Self-regulation failure: an overview.' *Psychological Inquiry*. v7(1):1–15. http://www.dartmouth. edu/~thlab/pubs/96_Baumeister_Heatherton_PI_7.pdf

7. Bossert-Zaudig S. et al. (1991) 'Hunger and appetite during visual perception of food in eating disorders.' *European Psychiatry*. v6 (5): 237–42 https://www.researchgate.net/publication/282493957_Hunger_and_ appetite_during_visual_perception_of_food_in_eating_disorders

8. Carver C. S., Scheier M. F. (1998) *On the Self-Regulation of Behavior.* New York: Cambridge University Press

9. Amitav C., Janiszewski C. (2004) 'The influence of generic advertising on brand preferences.' Journal of Consumer Research. v30(4):487– 502 http://warrington.ufl.edu/departments/mkt/docs/janiszewski/ InfluenceofGenericAdv.pdf

10. Alexander C., Gal D. (2010) 'Categorization effects in value judgments: averaging bias in evaluating combinations of vices and virtue.' *Journal of Marketing Research*, v47(4):738–47 http://journals.ama.org/doi/ abs/10.1509/jmkr.47.4.738

11. 'Why Food Companies Use Red Colors.' ColorSchemer | Instant Color Schemes n.p., 17 July 2007.

12. Boyatzis C. J., Varghese R. (1994) 'Children's emotional associations with colors.' *Journal of Genetic Psychology* v155(1):77–85 http://www. tandfonline.com/doi/abs/10.1080/00221325.1994.9914760

13. Chang W. L., Lin H. L. (2010) 'The impact of color traits on corporate branding.' *Afr. J Bus. Manage.* v4(15):3344–55 https://www.researchgate. net/publication/228370451_The_impact_of_color_traits_on_ corporate_branding

14. Clarke T., Costall A. (2008) 'The emotional connotations of color: a qualitative investigation.' *Color Research & Application.* v33(5):406–10 http://onlinelibrary.wiley.com/doi/10.1002/col.20435/abstract

15. Smith K. (2013) 'Blue packaging says healthy eating.' *Sensational Color*. http://www.sensationalcolor.com/business-of-color/product- packaging-colors/blue-packaging-healthy-1299#.Vt6kvlXcvIU

16. BBC One (2015) 'Tomorrow's Food Series One, Episode Two' http:// www.bing.com/videos/h?q=tomorrows+food+series+1+episode+1&vi

ew=detail&mid=8F56B155C779C1130D8E8F56B155C779C1130D8
E&FORM=VIRE

17. Wansink B., Chandon P. (2006) 'Can "low-fat" nutrition labels lead to obesity?.' *Journal of Marketing Research* v43(4):605–17 http://foodpsychology.cornell.edu/research/can-low-fat-nutrition-labels-lead-obesity

Chapter 5: Bad Halogens

1. Gold M. S., Pottash A. L. C., Extein I. (1981) 'Hypothyroidism and depression: evidence from complete thyroid function evaluation.' *Journal of the American Medical Association* (JAMA). v245(19).1919–22 http://jama.jamanetwork.com/article.aspx?articleid=375004

2. Radhakrishnan R. et al. (2013) 'Thyroid dysfunction in major psychiatric disorders in a hospital based sample.' *Indian Journal of Medical Research*. v138(6):888–93. http://www.ncbi.nlm.nih.gov/pmc/articles/PMC3978977/

3. Demartini B. et al. (2014) 'Depressive symptoms and major depressive disorder in patients affected by subclinical hypothyroidism: a cross-sectional study.' *Journal of Nervous and Mental Disease.* v202(8):603–7. http://www.ncbi.nlm.nih.gov/pubmed/25010109

4. Demartini B. et al. (2010) 'Prevalence of depression in patients affected by subclinical hypothyroidism.' *Panminerva medica.* v52(4):277–82. http://www.ncbi.nlm.nih.gov/pubmed/21183887

5. Grandjean P., Landrigan P. L. (2014) 'The Lancet Neurology,' v13(3) 330–8 http://www.thelancet.com/journals/laneur/article/PIIS1474-4422(13)70278-3/abstract

6. The 14 Nobel Prize Winning Scientists who oppose the fluoridation of drinking water 1) Adolf Butenandt (Chemistry, 1939) 2) Arvid Carlsson (Medicine, 2000) 3) Hans von Euler-Chelpin (Chemistry, 1929). 4) Walter Rudolf Hess (Medicine, 1949) 5) Corneille Jean-François Heymans (Medicine, 1938) 6) Sir Cyril Norman Hinshelwood (Chemistry, 1956) 7) Joshua Lederberg (Medicine, 1958) 8) William P. Murphy (Medicine, 1934) 9) Giulio Natta (1963 Nobel Prize in Chemistry) 10) Sir Robert Robinson (Chemistry, 1947) 11) Nikolay Semenov (Chemistry, 1956) 12) James B. Sumner (Chemistry, 1946) 13) Hugo Theorell (Medicine, 1955) 14) Artturi Virtanen (Chemistry, 1945)

7. Motl J., Siblerud R. L., Kienholz E. (1994) 'Psychometric evidence that mercury from silver dental fillings may be an etiological factor in depression, excessive anger and anxiety.' *Psychol Rep.* Feb v74(1):67–80. http://www.ncbi.nlm.nih.gov/pubmed/8153237

8.   Siblerud R. L. (1989) 'The relationship between mercury from dental amalgam and mental health.' *American Journal of Psychotherapy*. Oct v43(4):575-87. http://www.ncbi.nlm.nih.gov/pubmed/2618948

9.   Siblerud R. L., Kienholz E. (1994) 'Evidence that mercury from silver dental fillings may be an etiological factor in multiple sclerosis.' Journal? Mar v142(3):191–205. http://www.ncbi.nlm.nih.gov/pubmed/8191275

10. Barregard L., Sallsten G., Jarholm B. (1995) 'People with high mercury intake from their own dental amalgam fillings.' *Occup Environ Med*. Feb v52(2):124–8. http://www.ncbi.nlm.nih.gov/pubmed/7757165

11. Kingman A., Albertini T., Brown L. J. (1998) 'Mercury concentrations in urine and whole blood associated with amalgam exposure in a US military population.' *J Dent Res*. Mar v77(3):461–71. http://www.ncbi.nlm.nih.gov/pubmed/9496919

12. Yokoo E. M. et al. (2003) 'Low level methylmercury exposure affects neuropsychological function in adults.' *Environ Health*. Jun v2(8) http://www.ncbi.nlm.nih.gov/pmc/articles/PMC165591/

13. Yoshizawa K. et al. (2002) 'Mercury and the risk of coronary heart disease in men.' *N Engl J Med*. v347:1735–6. http://www.nejm.org/doi/full/10.1056/NEJMoa021437

14. CDC Centers for Disease Control and Prevention. 'Blood Mercury Levels in Young Children and Childbearing-aged Women–United States, 1999–2002 http://www.cdc.gov/mmwr/preview/mmwrhtml/mm5343a5.htm

15. National Research Council/National Academy of Sciences (2000) *Toxicological Effects of Methylmercury*. Washington DC: National Academy of Sciences Press http://www.nap.edu/read/9899/chapter/1

16. Lebel J. et al. (1998) 'Neurotoxic effects of low-level methylmercury contamination in the Amazonian Basin.' *Environ Res*. Oct v79(1):20–32. http://www.ncbi.nlm.nih.gov/pubmed/9756677

17. CDC Centers for Disease Control and Prevention (1999) 'Thimerosal in vaccines: a joint statement of the American Academy of Pediatrics and the Public Health Service.' *Morb Mortal Wkly Rep*. v48:563–5 http://www.cdc.gov/mmwr/preview/mmwrhtml/mm4826a3.htm

18. Midthun K. (2004) 'Thimerosal as a preservative in vaccines: an FDA perspective.' Presented 2004 in 'Mercury: Medical and Public Health Issues.' Tampa, Florida. 25–28 April

19. CDC Centers for Disease Control and Prevention (1996) 'Mercury poisoning associated with beauty cream–Texas, New Mexico, and California, 1995–1996.' *Morb Mortal Wkly Rep*. v45:400.

20. Saint-Phard D., Gonzalez P. G., Sherman P. (2004) 'Poster 88 unsuspected mercury toxicity linked to neurologic symptoms: A case series.' *Arch Phys Med Rehabil*. v85(9):E25. http://www.fda.gov/ohrms/dockets/dailys/04/sep04/092404/04d-0028-EC8-01.pdf

21. Cherian M. G. et al. (1978) 'Radioactive mercury distribution in

biological fluids and excretion in human subjects after inhalation of mercury vapor.' *Arch Environ Health.* May–Jun v33(3):109–14. http://www.ncbi.nlm.nih.gov/pubmed/686833

Chapter 6: Macronutrients vs Micronutrients

1. Khazan O. (2015) 'Why it was easier to be skinny in the 1980s.' *The Atlantic* http://www.theatlantic.com/health/archive/2015/09/why-it-was-easier-to-be-skinny-in-the-1980s/407974/

2. Sheridan K. (2015) 'ADHD Diagnoses Soar 43 Per cent in United States.' http://news.yahoo.com/adhd-diagnoses-soar-43-per cent-in-united-states-144844063.html?nf=1

3. Cordain L. et al. (2005) 'Origins and evolution of the Western diet: health implications for the 21st century.' *Am J Clin Nutr.* Feb v81(2):341–54 http://ajcn.nutrition.org/content/81/2/341.full

4. Leonard B., Maes M. (2012) 'Mechanistic explanations how cell-mediated immune activation, inflammation and oxidative and nitrosative stress pathways and their sequels and concomitants play a role in the pathophysiology of unipolar depression.' *Neurosci Biobehav Rev.* Feb v36(2):764–85. http://www.ncbi.nlm.nih.gov/pubmed/22197082

5. Moylan S. et al. (2013) 'The neuroprogressive nature of major depressive disorder: pathways to disease evolution and resistance, and therapeutic implications.' *Mol Psychiatry.* v18:595–606. http://www.nature.com/mp/journal/v18/n5/full/mp201233a.html

6. Maes M. et al. (2011) 'Depression's multiple comorbidities explained by (neuro)inflammatory and oxidative & nitrosative stress pathways.' *Neuro Endocrinol Lett.* v32(1):7–24. http://dro.deakin.edu.au/view/DU:30047558

7. Kubera M. et al. (2011) 'In animal models, psychosocial stress-induced (neuro)inflammation, apoptosis and reduced neurogenesis are associated to the onset of depression.' *Prog Neuropsychopharmacol Biol Psychiatry.* v35(3):744–59. http://www.sciencedirect.com/science/article/pii/S0278584610003465

8. Maes M. et al. (2012) 'New drug targets in depression: inflammatory, cell-mediated immune, oxidative and nitrosative stress, mitochondrial, antioxidant, and neuroprogressive pathways. And new drug candidates-Nrf2 activators and GSK-3 inhibitors.' *Inflammopharmacology.* v20(3):127–50. http://www.ncbi.nlm.nih.gov/pubmed/22271002

9. Hunt W. T. et al. (2010) 'Protection of cortical neurons from excitotoxicity by conjugated linoleic acid'. *J Neurochem.* Oct v115(1):123–30. http://www.ncbi.nlm.nih.gov/pubmed/20633209

10. 'USDA Revokes Grass Fed Label Standard' (2016) Morning Agclips website https://www.morningagclips.com/usda-revokes-grass-fed-label-standard/

11. Whitley A. (2010) 'The unpalatable truth about supermarket bread.' *Daily Mail* http://www.dailymail.co.uk/femail/food/article-1298227/Tescos-misleading-claims-bread-just-tip-iceberg.html

12. Mayo Clinic http://www.mayoclinic.org/drugs-supplements/omega-3-fatty-acids-fish-oil-alpha-linolenic-acid/dosing/hrb-20059372

13. Spencer B. (2015) 'Low-fat diets do NOT work: scientists cast doubt on years of health advice after concluding there is no evidence that reducing fat intake helps cut weight.' *Daily Mail* http://www.dailymail.co.uk/health/article-3296075/Trying-lose-weight-Ditch-low-fat-diet-Scientists-cast-doubt-years-health-advice-concluding-no-evidence-reducing-fat-intake-helps-cut-weight.html

14. The Health Editor (2015) 'The Surprising Link Between Carbs and Depression' http://news.health.com/2015/08/10/could-too-many-refined-carbs-make-you-depressed/

15. Malcolm L. and Willis O. (2015) 'Diet's Effects on the Brain Greater than Previously Thought' http://www.abc.net.au/radionational/programs/allinthemind/diet's-effects-on-the-brain-greater-than-previously-thought/6888576

16. Ruppel Shell E. (2015) 'Artificial sweeteners may change our gut bacteria in dangerous ways.' *Scientific American* http://www.scientificamerican.com/article/artificial-sweeteners-may-change-our-gut-bacteria-in-dangerous-ways/

17. Kovatsi L., Tsouggas M. (2014) 'The effect of oral aspartame administration on the balance of magnesium in the rat.' *Magnes Res* Sep v14(3):189-94. http://www.ncbi.nlm.nih.gov/pubmed/11599551

18. Newitz A. (2015) 'New Study Suggests Alzheimer's is Associated with Brain Fungus' http://gizmodo.com/new-study-suggests-alzheimers-is-associated-with-brain-1738788855

19. Thistlethwaite F. (2015) 'Nearly four MILLION Brits haven't drunk a glass of water in OVER a week.' *Express* http://www.express.co.uk/life-style/health/596507/Four-million-Brits-water-drink-over-week-hydration

20. Grossman E. (2015) 'We're flushing All These Antidepressants into Our Water.' How Big is the Problem? http://www.vox.com/2015/10/11/9489811/drugs-water-pollution

21. Macht H. (2015) 'The Link Between Diabetes, Pesticides and PCBs' http://www.endocrineweb.com/news/diabetes/17611-link-between-endocrine-disrupting-chemicals-diabetes

22. Weller C. (2014) 'Are ADHD, other mental disorders products of chemical exposure? Pesticides and fluoride among new risks.' *Medical Daily* http://www.medicaldaily.com/are-adhd-other-mental-disorders-products-chemical-exposure-pesticides-and-fluoride-among-new-risks

23. Blythman J. (2015) 'Why should I eat organic? You asked Google – here's the answer.' *The Guardian* http://www.theguardian.com/commentisfree/2015/oct/07/why-should-i-eat-organic-google

24. The Soil Association website http://www.soilassociation.org/whatisorganic/organicanimals

25. 'EWG's Dirty Dozen and Clean Fifteen Food Lists' http://www.ewg.org/foodnews/index.php

26. Pesticide Action Network UK (2013) 'Pesticide on a Plate' http://www.pan-uk.org/files/pesticides_on_a_plate_2013_final.pdf

27. Zahedi H. et al. (2014) 'Association between junk food consumption and mental health in a national sample of Iranian children and adolescents: the CASPIAN-IV study.' *Nutrition*. Nov–Dec v30(11–12):1391–7 http://www.ncbi.nlm.nih.gov/pubmed/25280418

28. Sánchez-Villegas A. et al. (2012) 'Fast-food and commercial baked goods consumption and the risk of depression.' *Public Health Nutr.* Mar v15(3):424–32 http://www.ncbi.nlm.nih.gov/pubmed/21835082

29. Daniel H. et al. (2014) 'High-fat diet alters gut microbiota physiology in mice.' *ISME J.* Feb v8(2):295–308 http://www.ncbi.nlm.nih.gov/pubmed/24030595

30. Aris A. (2011) 'Multiple toxins from GMOs detected in maternal and fetal blood.' *Reproductive Toxicology.* May v31(4):528–33 http://www.sciencedirect.com/science/article/pii/S0890623811000566

31. Spisák S. et al. (2013) 'Complete genes may pass from food to human blood *PLOS One*.' July

32. http://journals.plos.org/plosone/article?id=10.1371/journal.pone.0069805

33. Institute of Responsible Technology (IRT) Press Release (2013) 'Genetically Modified Foods Proposed as Trigger for Gluten Sensitivity' *IRT* http://responsibletechnology.org/media/images/content/Press_Release_Gluten_11_25.pdf

34. Séralini G. E. et al. (2012) 'Long term toxicity of a Roundup herbicide and a Roundup-tolerant genetically modified maize.' *Food Chem Toxicol.* Nov v50(11):4221–31. http://www.ncbi.nlm.nih.gov/pubmed/22999595

35. Thongprakaisang S. et al. (2013) 'Glyphosate induces human breast cancer cells growth via estrogen receptors.' *Food Chem Toxicol.* Sep v59:129–36 http://www.ncbi.nlm.nih.gov/pubmed/23756170

36. Samsel A., Seneff S. (2013) 'Glyphosate's suppression of cytochrome P450 enzymes and amino acid biosynthesis by the Gut microbiome: pathways to modern diseases.' *Entropy.* v15(4), 1416–63 http://www.mdpi.com/1099-4300/15/4/1416

37. Krüger M. et al. (2014) 'Detection of glyphosate residues in animals and humans.' *J Environ Anal Toxicol.* v4:2 http://www.omicsonline.org/open-access/detection-of-glyphosate-residues-in-animals-and-humans-2161-0525.1000210.pdf

38. Spisák S. et al. (2013) 'Complete genes may pass from food to human blood.' *PLOS One.* v8(7) http://journals.plos.org/plosone/article?id=10.1371/journal.pone.0069805

Chapter 8: Essential Supplements: 'The Big 4'

1. Fernandex C. (2015) 'Chimps detox too! Primates binge on mineral-rich clay to purify their bodies and boost their health.' *Daily Mail* http://www.dailymail.co.uk/sciencetech/article-3177679/Chimps-detox-Primates-binge-mineral-rich-clay-purify-bodies-boost-health.html

2. Institute of Medicine (1997) *Dietary Reference Intakes for Calcium, Phosphorus, Magnesium, Vitamin D, and Fluoride.* Washington, DC: National Academy Press. http://www.ncbi.nlm.nih.gov/books/NBK109825/

3. Altura B. M., Altura B. T. (2007) 'Magnesium: Forgotten mineral in cardiovascular biology and therogenesis, In *International Magnesium Symposium. New Perspectives in Magnesium Research.* London: Springer-Verlag, 239–60.

4. World Health Organization (2009) *Calcium and Magnesium in Drinking Water: Public health Significance.* Geneva: World Health Organization Press http://www.who.int/water_sanitation_health/publications/publication_9789241563550/en/

5. Pao E. M., Mickle S. J. (1981) 'Problem nutrients in the United States.' *Food Technology.* v35:58–79.

6. King D. E. et al. (2005) 'Dietary magnesium and C-reactive protein levels.' *Journal of the American College Of Nutrition.* Jun v24(3):166–71 http://www.anaboliclabs.com/User/Document/Articles/Magnesium/5.%20King,%20MAGnesium,%202005.pdf

7. Bohn T. (2008) 'Dietary factors influencing magnesium absorption in humans.' *Current Nutrition & Food Science.* v4(1):53–72. https://www.researchgate.net/publication/233603748_Dietary_Factors_Influencing_Magnesium_Absorption_in_Humans

8. McCarthy J., Kumar R. (1999) 'Divalent cation metabolism: magnesium', in Schrier R, series editor, *Atlas of Diseases of the Kidney.* Volume 1. Wiley-Blackwell 4.1-4.12.

9. Seelig M., Rosanoff A. (2003) *The Magnesium Factor.* New York: Avery

10. Dean C. (2007) *The Magnesium Miracle.* New York: Ballantine Books

11. Lieberman S., Bruning N. (2007) *The Real Vitamin & Mineral Book.* New York: Avery,

12. Chouinard G. et al. (1990) 'A pilot study of magnesium aspartate hydrochloride (Magnesiocard®) as a mood stabilizer for rapid cycling bipolar affective disorder patients.' *Progress in Neuro-Psychopharmacology and Biological Psychiatry.* v14(2):171–80. http://www.sciencedirect.com/science/article/pii/0278584690900993

13. Heiden A. et al. (1999) 'Treatment of severe mania with intravenous

magnesium sulphate as a supplementary therapy.' *Psychiatry Research.* Dec v89(3):239–46. http://www.ncbi.nlm.nih.gov/pubmed/10708270

14. Birch E. E. et al. (2000) 'A randomized controlled trial of early dietary supply of long-chain polyunsaturated fatty acids and mental development in term infants.' *Developmental Medicine and Child Neurology.* Mar v42(3):174–81 http://www.ncbi.nlm.nih.gov/pubmed/10755457

15. Glomset J. A. (2006) 'Role of docosahexaenoic acid in neuronal plasma membranes.' *Sci STKE.* v321 http://www.ncbi.nlm.nih.gov/pubmed/16467193

16. Litman B. J. et al. (2001) 'The role of docosahexaenoic acid containing phospholipids in modulating G protein-coupled signaling pathways: visual transduction.' *J Mol. Neurosci.* v16(2–3):237–42 http://www.ncbi.nlm.nih.gov/pubmed/11478379

17. O'Brien J. S., Sampson L. (1965) 'Fatty acid and fatty aldehyde composition of the major brain lipids in normal human gray matter, white matter, and myelin.' *J Lipid Res.* v6:545–51. http://www.jlr.org/content/6/4/545.short

18. Salem N. Jr et al. (2001) 'Mechanism of action of docosahexaenoic acid in the nervous system.' *Lipids.* v36(9):945–59. http://www.ncbi.nlm.nih.gov/pubmed/11724467

19. SanGiovanni J. P., Chew E. Y. (2005) 'The role of omega-3 long-chain polyunsaturated fatty acids in health and disease of the retina.' *Progress in Retinal and Eye Research.* v24(1):87–138. http://www.sciencedirect.com/science/article/pii/S1350946204000527

20. Stilwell W., Wassall S. R. (2003) 'Docosahexaenoic acid: membrane properties of a unique fatty acid.' *Chemistry and Physics of Lipids.* v126(1):1–27. http://www.sciencedirect.com/science/article/pii/S0009308403001014

21. Svennerholm L. (1968) 'Distribution and fatty acid composition of phosphoglycerides in normal human brain.' *J Lipid Res.* Sep v9(5):570–9. http://www.ncbi.nlm.nih.gov/pubmed/4302302

22. Youdin K. A. et al. (2000) 'Essential fatty acids and the brain: possible health implications.' *Int. J Neurosci.* Jul–Aug v18(4–5):383–99. http://www.ncbi.nlm.nih.gov/pubmed/10817922

23. Clayton E. H. et al. (2009) 'Reduced mania and depression in juvenile bipolar disorder associated with long-chain omega-3 polyunsaturated fatty acid supplementation.' *Eur J Clin Nutr.* Jan v63(8):1037–40. http://www.nature.com/ejcn/journal/v63/n8/full/ejcn200881a.html

24. Ross B. M., Maxwell R., Glen I. (2010) 'Increased breath ethane levels in medicated patients with schizophrenia and bipolar disorder are unrelated to erythrocyte omega-3 fatty acid abundance.' *Prog Neuropsychopharmacol Biol Psychiatry.* Mar v35(2):446–53

25. http://www.ncbi.nlm.nih.gov/pubmed/21115087

26. Osher Y., Bersudsky Y., Belmaker R. H. (2005) 'Omega-3

eicosapentaenoic acid in bipolar depression: report of a small open-label study.' *J Clin Psychiatry*. Jun v66(6):726–29. http://www.ncbi.nlm.nih.gov/pubmed/15960565

27. Noaghiul S., Hibbeln J. R. (2003) 'Cross-national comparisons of seafood consumption and rates of bipolar disorders.' *Am J Psychiatry*. Dec v160(12):2222–7. http://www.ncbi.nlm.nih.gov/pubmed/14638594

28. Behzadi A. H. et al. (2009) 'Folic acid efficacy as an alternative drug added to sodium calproate in the treatment of acute phase of mania in bipolar disorder: a double blind randomized controlled trial.' *Acta Psychiatr Scand*. Dec v120(6):441–5 http://www.ncbi.nlm.nih.gov/pubmed/19392814

29. Dias V. V. et al. (2009) 'Serum homocysteine levels and cognitive functioning in euthymic bipolar patients.' *J Affect Disord*. v113(3):285–90. http://www.ncbi.nlm.nih.gov/pubmed/18579214

30. Osher Y. et al. (2008) 'Neuropsychological correlates of homocysteine levels in euthymic bipolar patients.' *J of affective disorders*. v105(1):229–33. https://www.researchgate.net/publication/6340661_Neuropsychological_correlates_of_homocysteine_levels_in_euthymic_bipolar_patients

31. Reynolds E. H. (1968) 'Mental effects of anticonvulsants, and folic acid metabolism.' *Brain*. v91(2):197–214. https://www.researchgate.net/publication/17463993_Mental_Effects_of_Anticonvulsants_and_Folic_Acid_Metabolism

32. Botez M. I., Reynolds E. H., editor (1979) *Folic Acid in Neurology, Psychiatry and Internal Medicine*. New York: Raven

33. Reynolds E. H. (2002) 'Benefits and risks of folic acid to the nervous system.' *J Neurol Neurosurg Psychiatry*. v72(5):567–71. https://www.researchgate.net/publication/11397409_Benefits_and_risks_of_folic_acid_to_the_nervous_system

34. Shorvon S. D. et al. (1980) 'The neuropsychiatry of megaloblastic anaemia.' *Br Med J*. v281:1036–142. http://www.ncbi.nlm.nih.gov/pmc/articles/PMC1714413/

35. Clarke R. et al. (1998) 'Folate, vitamin B12, and serum total homocysteine levels in confirmed Alzheimer disease.' *Arch Neurol*. v55(11):1449–55. http://www.ncbi.nlm.nih.gov/pubmed/9823829

36. Selhub J. et al. (2000) 'B vitamins, homocysteine and neuro cognitive function in the elderly.' *Am J Clin Nutr*. v71(suppl):S614–S620. http://ajcn.nutrition.org/content/71/2/614s.long

37. Snowdon D. A. et al. (2000) 'Serum folate and the severity of atrophy of the neocortex in Alzheimer disease: findings from the nun study.' *Am J Clin Nutr*. v71(4):993–8. http://www.ncbi.nlm.nih.gov/pubmed/10731508

38. Seshadri S. et al. (2002) 'Plasma homocysteine as a risk factor for dementia and Alzheimer's disease.' *N Engl J Med*. v346(7):476–83. http://www.ncbi.nlm.nih.gov/pubmed/11844848

39. Botez M. I. et al. (1977) 'Folate-responsive neurological and mental disorders: report of 16 cases.' *Eur Neurol.* v16(1–6):230–46. http://www.karger.com/Article/Abstract/114904

40. Reynolds E. H., Rothfeld P., Pincus J. (1973) 'Neurological disease associated with folate deficiency.' *Br Med J.* v2(5863):398–400. http://www.ncbi.nlm.nih.gov/pmc/articles/PMC1589924/

41. Carney M. W. P. et al. (1990) 'Red cell folate concentrations in psychiatric patients.' *J Affect Disord.* v19(3):207–13. http://www.jad-journal.com/article/0165-0327(90)90093-N/pdf

42. Reynolds E. H. et al. (1970) 'Folate deficiency in depressive illness.' *Br J Psychiatry.* v117(538):287–92. https://www.researchgate.net/publication/51271413_Folate_deficiency_in_depressive_illness

43. Bottiglieri T. et al. (2000) 'Homocysteine, folate, methylation and monoamine metabolism in depression.' *J Neurol Neurosurg Psychiatry.* v69(2):228–32. http://www.ncbi.nlm.nih.gov/pubmed/10896698

44. Coppen A., Chaudhry S., Swade C. (1986) Folic acid enhances lithium prophylaxis. *J Affect Disord.* v10(1):9–13. http://www.ncbi.nlm.nih.gov/pubmed/2939126

45. Coppen A., Bailey J. (2000) 'Enhancement of the antidepressant action of fluoxetine by folic acid: a randomised, placebo controlled trial.' *J Affect Disord.* v60(2):121–30. http://www.jad-journal.com/article/S0165-0327(00)00153-1/abstract

46. Godfrey P. S. A. et al. (1990) 'Enhancement of recovery from psychiatric illness by methyl folate.' *Lancet.* v336(8712):392–5. http://www.ncbi.nlm.nih.gov/pubmed/1974941

47. Bottiglieri T., Reynolds E. H., Laundy M. (2000) 'Folate in CSF and age.' *J Neurol Neurosurg Psychiatry.* v69(4):562. https://www.researchgate.net/publication/12148074_Folate_in_CSF_and_age

48. Wang H-X. et al. (2001) 'Vitamin B12 and folate in relation to the development of Alzheimer's disease.' *Neurology.* v56(9):1188–94. http://www.neurology.org/content/56/9/1188.1.abstract

49. Passeri M. et al. (1993) 'Oral 5-methyltetrahydrofolic acid in senile organic mental disorders with depression: results of a double-blind multicenter study.' *Aging Clin Exp Res.* v5(1):63–71. http://www.ncbi.nlm.nih.gov/pubmed/8257478

50. Goodwin J. S., Goodwin J. M., Garry P. J. (1983) 'Association between nutritional status and cognitive functioning in a healthy elderly population.' *JAMA.* v249(21):2917–21. http://jama.jamanetwork.com/article.aspx?articleid=386944

51. La Rue A. et al. (1997) 'Nutritional status and cognitive functioning in a normally aging sample: a six year reassessment.' *Am J Clin Nutr.* v65(1):20–9. http://intl-ajcn.nutrition.org/content/65/1/20.abstract

52. Riggs K. M. et al. (1996) 'Relations of vitamin B12, vitamin B6, folate and homocysteine to cognitive performance in the normative

aging study.' *Am J Clin Nutr.* v63(3):306–14. http://ajcn.nutrition.org/content/63/3/306.short?related-urls=yes&legid=ajcn;63/3/306

53. Wahlin T. B. R. et al. (2001) 'The influence of serum vitamin B12 and folate status on cognitive functioning in very old age.' *Biol Psychol.* v56(3):247–65. http://www.sciencedirect.com/science/article/pii/S0301051101000795

54. Reynolds E. H., Carney M. W. P., Toone B. K. (1984) 'Methylation and mood.' *Lancet.* V2(8396):196–8. http://www.ncbi.nlm.nih.gov/pubmed/6146753

55. Bottiglieri T. et al. (1990) 'Cerebrospinal fluid S-adenosylmethionine in depression and dementia: effects of treatment with parenteral and oral S-adenosyl methionine.' *J Neurol Neurosurg Psychiatry.* v53(12):1096–8. http://www.ncbi.nlm.nih.gov/pmc/articles/PMC488323/

56. Goggans F. (1984) 'A case of mania secondary to vitamin B12 deficiency.' *Am J Psychiatry.* Feb v141(2):300–1. http://ajp.psychiatryonline.org/doi/10.1176/ajp.141.2.300

57. Fafouti M. et al. (2002) 'Mood disorder with mixed features due to vitamin B12 and folate deficiency.' *General Hospital Psychiatry.* Mar–Apr v24(2):106–09. http://www.sciencedirect.com/science/article/pii/S0163834301001815

58. Demirhan O., Tastemir D., Sertdemir Y. (2009) 'The expression of folate sensitive fragile sites in patients with bipolar disorder.' *Yonsei Med J.* Feb v50(1):137–41.http://www.ncbi.nlm.nih.gov/pmc/articles/PMC2649857/

59. McNamara R. K. (2010) 'DHA deficiency and prefrontal cortex neuropathology in recurrent affective disorders.' *The Journal of Nutrition.* Apr v140(4):864–8. http://www.ncbi.nlm.nih.gov/pmc/articles/PMC2838627/

60. Hamazaki K., Choi K. H., Kim H-Y. (2010) 'Phospholipid profile in the postmortem hippocampus of patients with schizophrenia and bipolar disorder: no changes in docosahexaenoic acid species.' *Journal of Psychiatric Research.* v44(11):688–93. http://www.ncbi.nlm.nih.gov/pubmed/20056243

61. Prabhakar K. R. et al. (2003) 'Decreased antioxidant enzymes and membrane essential polyunsaturated fatty acids in schizophrenic and bipolar mood disorder patients.' *Psychiatry Research* v121(2):109–22. http://www.psy-journal.com/article/S0165-1781(03)00220-8/abstract

62. Porter Phillips J. G. (1910) 'The treatment of melancholia by the lactic acid bacillus.' *British Journal of Psychiatry.* Jul v56(234):422–NP http://bjp.rcpsych.org/content/56/234/422.short

63. Steenbergen L. et al. (2015) 'A randomised controlled trial to test the effect of multispecies probiotics on cognitive reactivity to sad mood.' *Brain, Behaviour and Immunity.* Aug v:258–64 http://www.sciencedirect.com/science/article/pii/S0889159115000884

64. Ventek Rao A. et al. (2009) 'A randomised, double-blind, placebo

controlled study of a probiotic in emotional symptoms of chronic fatigue syndrome.' *Gut Pathogens.* v1(6) http://gutpathogens.biomedcentral. com/articles/10.1186/1757-4749-1-6

65. Bested A. C. et al. (2013) 'Intestinal microbiota, probiotics and mental health.' *Gut Pathogens.* v5(3) http://www.ncbi.nlm.nih.gov/pmc/articles/ PMC3601973/

66. Selhub E. M. (2014) 'Fermented foods, microbiota, and mental health.' *Journal of Physiological Anthropology.* v33(1) 2 http://www.ncbi.nlm.nih. gov/pmc/articles/PMC3904694/

67. Messaoudi M. et al. (2011) 'Beneficial psychological effects of a probiotic formulation in healthy human volunteers.' *Gut Microbes.* Jul–Aug v2(4)256–61. http://www.ncbi.nlm.nih.gov/pubmed/21983070

Chapter 9: Additional Supplements to Consider

1. Hoogendijk W. J. et al. (2008) 'Depression is associated with decreased 25-Hydroxyvitamin D and increased parathyroid hormone levels in older adults.' *Arch Gen Psychiatry.* May v65(5):508–12. http://www.ncbi. nlm.nih.gov/pubmed/18458202

2. Reinhold V. et al. (2004) 'Randomized comparison of the effects of the vitamin D_3 adequate intake versus 100 mcg (4000IU) per day on biochemical responses and the wellbeing of patients.' *Nutrition Journal* v3(8) http://www.ncbi.nlm.nih.gov/pmc/articles/PMC506781/

3. Shipowick C. D. et al. (2009) 'Vitamin D and depressive symptoms in women during the winter: a pilot study.' *Appl Nurs Res.* Aug v22(3):221–5. http://www.ncbi.nlm.nih.gov/pubmed/19616172

4. McGrath J. et al. (2003) 'Low maternal vitamin D as a risk factor for schizophrenia: a pilot study using banked sera.' Sep v63(1–2):73–8

5. http://www.sciencedirect.com/science/article/pii/ S0920996402004358

6. Reinhold V. et al. (2007) 'The urgent need to recommend an intake of vitamin D that is effective.' *Am J Clin Nutr* (Paper jointly written by 15 specialists) http://ajcn.nutrition.org/content/85/3/649.full

7. Cherniack E. P. et al. (2009) 'Some new food for thought: the role of vitamin D in the mental health of older adults.' *Current Psychiatry Reports.* v11:12 http://link.springer.com/article/10.1007/s11920-009-0003-3

8. P.J., J. P. (2014) 'A statistical error in the estimation of the recommended dietary allowance for vitamin D.' *Nutrients.* Oct v6(10):4472–5. http:// www.ncbi.nlm.nih.gov/pmc/articles/PMC4210929/

9. Mah E. et al. (2015) 'α-Tocopherol bioavailability is lower in adults with metabolic syndrome regardless of dairy fat co-ingestion: a randomized, double-blind, crossover trial.' *Am J Clin Nutr.* Nov v102(5):1070–80 http://ajcn.nutrition.org/content/102/5/1070

10. Jackson Roberts II L. et al. (2007) 'The relationship between dose of

vitamin E and suppression of oxidative stress in humans.' *Free Radic Biol Med.* Nov v43(10):1388–93. http://www.ncbi.nlm.nih.gov/pmc/articles/PMC2072864/

11. Pace A. et al. (2010) 'Vitamin E neuroprotection for cisplatin neuropathy: a randomized, placebo-controlled trial.' *Neurology.* Mar v74(9):762–6 http://www.ncbi.nlm.nih.gov/pubmed/20194916

12. Malafa M. P., Neitzel L. T. (2000) 'Vitamin E succinate promotes breast cancer tumor dormancy.' *J Surg Res.* Sep v93(1):163–70 http://www.journalofsurgicalresearch.com/article/S0022-4804(00)95948-1/abstract

13. Mangialasche F., Klvipelto P. et al. (2010) 'High plasma levels of vitamin E forms and reduced Alzheimer's disease risk in advanced age.' *J Alzheimers Dis.* v20(4):1029–37. http://www.ncbi.nlm.nih.gov/pubmed/20413888

14. Masaki K. H., Losonczy K. G., Izmirlian G. (2000) 'Association of vitamin E and C supplement use with cognitive function and dementia in elderly men.' *Neurology.* v54(6):1265–72. http://www.neurology.org/content/54/6/1265.short

15. Mangialasche F. et al. (2012) 'Tocopherols and tocotrienols plasma levels are associated with cognitive impairment.' *Neurobiol Aging.* Oct v33(10):2282–90. http://www.ncbi.nlm.nih.gov/pubmed/22192241

16. Conner T. S., Richardson A. C., Miller J. C. (2015) 'Optimal serum selenium concentrations are associated with lower depressive symptoms and negative mood among young Adults.' *J Nutr.* v145(1)59–65 http://jn.nutrition.org/content/145/1/59.abstract?etoc

17. Rayman M. P. (1997) 'Dietary selenium: time to act.' *British Medical Journal.* 314: 387–8. http://epubs.surrey.ac.uk/185985/3/BMJ editorial1997.pdf

18. Jackson M. J., Broome C. S. and McArdle F. (2003) 'Marginal dietary selenium intakes in the UK: are there functional consequences?' *J. Nutr* v133(5) 15575–95 http://jn.nutrition.org/content/133/5/1557S.full

19. Sneddon A. (2012) 'Selenium nutrition and its impact on health.' Food and Health Innovation Service https://www.abdn.ac.uk/rowett/documents/selenium_and_health_august_2012.pdf

20. Benton D. (2002) 'Selenium intake, mood and other aspects of psychological functioning.' *Nutritional Neuroscience.* Dec v5(6):363–74 http://www.ncbi.nlm.nih.gov/pubmed/12509066?dopt=Abstract

21. Mokhber N. et al. (2011) 'Effect of supplementation with selenium on postpartum depression: a randomized double-blind placebo-controlled trial.' *Journal of Maternal-Fetal and Neonatal Medicine.* Jan v24(1):104–8. http://www.ncbi.nlm.nih.gov/pubmed/20528216

22. Sher L. (2001) 'Role of thyroid hormones in the effects of selenium on mood, behavior, and cognitive function.' *Medical Hypotheses.* Oct v57(4): 480–3 http://www.medical-hypotheses.com/article/S0306-9877.7%2801%2991369-6/abstract

23. Sher L. (2008) 'Depression and suicidal behavior in alcohol abusing adolescents: possible role of selenium deficiency.' *Minerva Pediatrica.* Apr v60(2):201–9. http://www.ncbi.nlm.nih.gov/pubmed/18449137

24. Combet E. et al. (2014) 'Low-level seaweed supplementation improves iodine status in iodine-insufficient women.' *Br J Nutr.* Sep v112(05):753–61 http://www.ncbi.nlm.nih.gov/pubmed/25006699

25. Wilcox M. D. et al. (2014) 'The modulation of pancreatic lipase activity by alginates.' *Food Chemistry.* Mar v146:479–84. http://www.ncbi.nlm.nih.gov/pubmed/24176371

26. Grønli O. et al. (2013) 'Zinc deficiency is common in several psychiatric disorders.' *PLOS One* v8(12):e82793. http://www.ncbi.nlm.nih.gov/pubmed/24367556

27. Maxwell C., Volpe S. L. (2007) 'Effect of zinc supplementation on thyroid hormone function: a case study of two college females.' *Ann Nutr Metab.* v51(2):188–94. http://www.ncbi.nlm.nih.gov/pubmed/17541266

28. Betsy A., Binitha M., Sarita S. (2013) 'Zinc deficiency associated with hypothyroidism: an overlooked cause of severe alopecia.' *Int J Trichology.* Jan–Mar v5(1):40–2. http://www.ncbi.nlm.nih.gov/pubmed/23960398

29. Ertek S. et al. (2010) 'Relationship between serum zinc levels, thyroid hormones and thyroid volume following successful iodine supplementation.' Jul–Sep v9(3):263–8. http://www.ncbi.nlm.nih.gov/pubmed/20688624

30. NEDA 2015 Annual Report https://www.nationaleatingdisorders.org/annualreport/2015/downloads/NEDA-Annual-Report-2015.pdf

31. Humphries L. et al. (1989) 'Zinc deficiency and eating disorders.' *J Clin Psychiatry.* Dec v50(12):456–9. http://www.ncbi.nlm.nih.gov/pubmed/260006

32. Szewczyk B. et al. (2010) 'The involvement of NMDA and AMPA receptors in the mechanism of antidepressant-like action of zinc in the forced swim test.' *Amino Acids.* Sep v39(1):205–17. https://www.researchgate.net/publication/40444076_The_involvement_of_NMDA_and_AMPA_receptors_in_the_mechanism_of_antidepressant-like_action_of_zinc_in_the_forced_swim_test

33. Cope E. C., Levenson C. W. (2010) 'Role of zinc in the development and treatment of mood disorders.' *Curr Opin Clin Nutr Metab Care.* Nov v13(6):685–9 http://www.ncbi.nlm.nih.gov/pubmed/20689416

34. D. H. et al. (2011) 'Polychlorinated biphenyls and organochlorine pesticides in plasma predict development of Type 2 diabetes in the Elderly.' *Diabetes Care Journal.* Aug v34(8):1778–84. http://www.ncbi.nlm.nih.gov/pmc/articles/PMC3142022/

35. Lee D. H. et al. (2016) 'Association between background exposure to organochlorine pesticides and the risk of cognitive impairment: a prospective study that accounts for weight change.' *Environment*

International, Apr–May v89–90:179–184 http://www.sciencedirect.com/science/article/pii/S0160412016300265

36. Mizoguchi T. et al. (2008) 'Nutrigenomic studies of effects of chlorella on subjects with high-risk factors for lifestyle-related disease.' *Journal of Medicinal Food*. Sep v11(3): 395–404. http://rawganik.com/studies/chlorgener.pdf

37. Horikoshi T., Nakajima A., Sakaguch T. (1979) 'Uptake of uranium by various cell fractions of chlorella regularis.' *Radioisotopes*. 28(8):485–8 https://www.researchgate.net/publication/22598923_Uptake_of_Uranium_by_Various_Cell_Fractions_of_Chlorella_regularis

38. Merchant R. E., Carmack C. A., Wise C. M. (2000) 'Nutritional supplementation with chlorella pyrenoidosa for patients with fibromyalgia syndrome.' *Phytother. Res.* v14:167–73. https://www.deepdyve.com/lp/wiley/nutritional-supplementation-with-chlorella-pyrenoidosa-for-patients-751JE7iv4c

39. Pore R. S. (1984) 'Detoxification of chlordecone poisoned rats with chlorella and chlorella-derived sporopollenin.' *Drug Chem Toxicol.* v7(1):57– 71 http://www.ncbi.nlm.nih.gov/pubmed/6202479

40. Morita K. et al. (1999) 'Chlorella accelerates dioxin excretion in rats.' *J Nutr.* Sep v129(9):1731–6, http://jn.nutrition.org/content/129/9/1731.

41. Konishi F. et al. (1996) 'Protective effect of an acidic glycoprotein obtained from culture of Chlorella vulgaris against myelosuppression by 5-fluorouracil.' *Cancer Immunil Innumother.* Jun v42(5):268–74, http://www.ncbi.nlm.nih.gov/pubmed/8706047

42. Mani U. V., Desai S. and Iyer U. (2000) 'Studies on the long-term effect of spirulina supplementation on serum lipid profile and glycated proteins in NIDDM patients.' *J Nutraceuticals Functional Med Foods.* v2(3):25–32 http://www.tandfonline.com/doi/abs/10.1300/J133v02n03_03?journalCode=ijds19

43. Gray A. M., Flatt P. R. (1999) 'Insulin-releasing and insulin-like activity of the traditional anti-diabetic plant Coriandrum sativum (coriander).' *Br J Nutr.* Mar v81(3):203–9. http://journals.cambridge.org/download.php?file=%2FBJN%2FBJN81_03%2FS0007114599000392a.pdf&code=2d6b77b6d5c3a8691339879b90c07d0c

44. Cioanca O. et al. (2013) 'Cognitive-enhancing and antioxidant activities of inhaled coriander volatile oil in amyloid β(1-42) rat model of Alzheimer's disease.' *Physiol Behav.* Aug v120:193–202. http://www.ncbi.nlm.nih.gov/pubmed/23958472

45. Baser K. H. (2008) 'Biological and pharmacological activities of carvacrol and carvacrol bearing essential oils.' *Curr Pharm Des.* v14(29):3106–19. http://www.ncbi.nlm.nih.gov/pubmed/19075694

46. Arunasree K. M. (2010) 'Anti-proliferative effects of carvacrol on a human metastatic breast cancer cell line, MDA-MB 231.' *Phytomedicine.* Jul v17(8-9):581–8. http://www.ncbi.nlm.nih.gov/pubmed/20096548

47. El Babili F. et al. (2011) 'Oregano: chemical analysis and evaluation of its antimalarial, antioxidant, and cytotoxic activities.' *J Food Sci.* Apr v76(3):C512-8. http://www.ncbi.nlm.nih.gov/pubmed/21535822

48. LIU Brooklyn Press Release (2012) 'LIU STUDY: Component in Oregano Kills Prostate Cancer Cells.' http://www.liu.edu/Brooklyn/ About/News/Campus-Press-Releases/2012/April/BK-PR-Apr25-2012

49. Andersen A. (2006) 'Final report on the safety assessment of sodium p-chloro-m-cresol, p-chloro-m-cresol, chlorothymol, mixed cresols, m-cresol, o-cresol, p-cresol, isopropyl cresols, thymol, o-cymen-5-ol, and carvacrol.' *Int J Toxicol.* v6(25 Suppl 1):29–127. http://ijt.sagepub.com/ content/25/1_suppl/29.abstract

50. Ozkan A., Erdogan A. (2012) 'A comparative study of the antioxidant/ prooxidant effects of carvacrol and thymol at various concentrations on membrane and DNA of parental and drug resistant H1299 cells.' *Nat Prod Commun.* Dec v7(12):1557–60. http://www.ncbi.nlm.nih.gov/ pubmed/23413548

51. Liang W. Z. et al. (2013) 'The mechanism of carvacrol-evoked [Ca2+] i rises and non-Ca2+-triggered cell death in OC2 human oral cancer cells.' *Toxicology.* Jan v303:152–61. http://www.ncbi.nlm.nih.gov/ pubmed/23146755

52. Liang W. Z., Lu C. H. (2012) 'Carvacrol-induced [Ca2+]i rise and apoptosis in human glioblastoma cells.' *Life Sci.* May v90(17–18):703–11. http://www.sciencedirect.com/science/article/pii/ S0024320512001506

53. Lu Y., Wu C. (2010) 'Reduction of Salmonella enterica contamination on grape tomatoes by washing with thyme oil, thymol, and carvacrol as compared with chlorine treatment.' *J Food Prot.* Dec v73(12):2270–5. http://www.ncbi.nlm.nih.gov/pubmed/21219747

54. Obaidat M. M., Frank J. F. (2009) 'Inactivation of Salmonella and Escherichia coli O157:H7 on sliced and whole tomatoes by allyl isothiocyanate, carvacrol, and cinnamaldehyde in vapor phase. *J Food Prot.* Feb v72(2):315-24. http://www.medscape.com/medline/ abstract/19350975

55. van Alphen L. B. et al. (2012) 'The natural antimicrobial carvacrol inhibits Campylobacter jejuni motility and infection of epithelial cells.' PLOS One. v7(9):e45343. http://www.ncbi.nlm.nih.gov/pmc/articles/ PMC3458047/

56. Upadhyay A. et al. (2012) 'Plant-derived antimicrobials reduce Listeria monocytogenes virulence factors in vitro, and down-regulate expression of virulence genes.' *Int J Food Microbiol.* Jun v157(1):88–94. http://www. sciencedirect.com/science/article/pii/S016816051200222X?np=y

57. Ravishankar S. et al. (2010) 'Carvacrol and cinnamaldehyde inactivate antibiotic-resistant Salmonella enterica in buffer and on celery and oysters.' *J Food Prot.* Feb v73(2):234–40. http://www.ncbi.nlm.nih.gov/pubmed/20132667

58. Marcos-Arias C. et al. (2011) 'In vitro activities of natural products against oral Candida isolates from denture wearers.' *BMC Complement Altern Med.* Nov v11:119. http://www.ncbi.nlm.nih.gov/pmc/articles/PMC3258290/

59. Kulisi T. et al. (2007) 'The effects of essential oils and aqueous tea infusions of oregano (Origanum vulgare L. spp. hirtum), thyme (Thymus vulgaris L.) and wild thyme (Thymus serpyllum L.) on the copper-induced oxidation of human low-density lipoproteins.' *Int J Food Sci Nutr.* Mar v58(2):87–93. http://www.ncbi.nlm.nih.gov/pubmed/17469764

60. Kemertelidze E. et al. (2012) 'Saturin – effective vegetative remedy in treatment of type 2 diabetes mellitus.' *Georgian Med News.* Feb (203):47–52. http://www.ncbi.nlm.nih.gov/pubmed/22466541

61. Hotta M. et al. (2010) 'Carvacrol, a component of thyme oil, activates PPARalpha and gamma and suppresses COX-2 expression.' *J Lipid Res.* Jan 51(1):132–9. http://www.ncbi.nlm.nih.gov/pubmed/19578162

62. Desai M. A. et al. (2012) 'Reduction of Listeria monocytogenes biofilms on stainless steel and polystyrene surfaces by essential oils.' *J Food Prot.* Jul v75(7):1332–7. http://www.ncbi.nlm.nih.gov/pubmed/22980020

63. Sato K., Krist S., Buchbauer G. (2007) 'Antimicrobial effect of vapours of geraniol, (R)-(-)-linalool, terpineol, gamma-terpinene and 1,8-cineole on airborne microbes using an airwasher.' *Flavour & Fragrance Journal.* v22(5):435–7 http://onlinelibrary.wiley.com/doi/10.1002/ffj.1818/abstract

64. Santos F. A., Rao V. S. (2000) 'Antiinflammatory and antinociceptive effects of 1,8-cineole a terpenoid oxide present in many plant essential oils.' *Phytotherapy Research.* v14(4):240–4 http://www.ncbi.nlm.nih.gov/pubmed/10861965

65. Liapi C. et al. (2007) 'Antinociceptive properties of 1,8-cineole and beta-pinene, from the essential oil of Eucalyptus camaldulensis leaves, in rodents.' *Planta Medica.* v73(12):1247–54 http://www.ncbi.nlm.nih.gov/pubmed/17893834

66. Pattnaik S. et al. (1997) 'Antibacterial and antifungal activity of aromatic constituents of essential oils.' *Microbios.* v89(358):39–46 http://www.ncbi.nlm.nih.gov/pubmed/9218354

67. Carson C. F., Mee B. J., Riley T. V. (2002) 'Mechanism of action of Melaleuca alternifolia (tea tree) oil on Staphylococcus aureus determined by time-kill, lysis, leakage, and salt tolerance assays and electron microscopy.' *Antimicrobial Agents and Chemotherapy.* v46(6):1914–20 http://aac.asm.org/content/46/6/1914.full

68. Juergens U. R. et al. (2003) 'Anti-inflammatory activity of 1,8 cineole

(eucalpytol) in bronchial asthma: a double blind, placebo controlled trial.' *Respiratory Medicine.* v97(3):250–6

69. Juergens U. R. et al. (2004) 'Inhibitory activity of 1,8-cineol (eucalyptol) on cytokine production in cultured human lymphocytes and monocytes.' *Pulm Pharmacol Ther.* v17(5):281–7 http://www.ncbi.nlm.nih.gov/pubmed/15477123

70. Santos F. A. et al. (2004) '1,8-Cineole (eucalyptol), a monoterpene oxide attenuates the colonic damage in rats on acute TNBS-colitis.' *Food & Chemical Toxicology.* Apr v42(2):579–84 http://www.ncbi.nlm.nih.gov/pubmed/15019181

71. Nascimento N. R. et al. (2009) '1,8-Cineole induces relaxation in rat and guinea-pig airway smooth muscle.' *Journal of Pharmacy & Pharmacology.* Mar v61(3):361–6 http://www.ncbi.nlm.nih.gov/pubmed/19222909

72. Coelho-de-Souza L. N. et al. (2005) 'Relaxant effects of the essential oil of Eucalyptus tereticornis and its main constituent 1,8-cineole on guinea-pig tracheal smooth muscle.' *Planta Medica.* Dec v71(12):1173–5 http://www.ncbi.nlm.nih.gov/pubmed/16395658

73. Bastos V. P. et al. (2009) 'Inhibitory effect of 1,8-cineole on guinea-pig airway challenged with ovalbumin involves a preferential action on electromechanical coupling.' *Clinical & Experimental Pharmacology & Physiology.* Nov v36(11):1120–6 http://onlinelibrary.wiley.com/doi/10.1111/j.1440-1681.2009.05189.x/abstract

74. Kako H. et al. (2008) 'Effects of direct exposure of green odour components on dopamine release from rat brain striatal slices and PC12 cells.' *Brain Res Bull.* Mar v75(5):706–12 http://www.ncbi.nlm.nih.gov/pubmed/18355650

75. Lahlou S. et al. (2002) 'Cardiovascular effects of 1,8 cineole, a terpenoid oxide present in many plant essential oils, in normotensive rats.' *Can J Physiol Pharmacol.* Dec v80(12):1125–31 http://www.ncbi.nlm.nih.gov/pubmed/12564637

76. Pinto N. V. et al. (2009) 'Endothelium-dependent vasorelaxant effects of the essential oil from aerial parts of Alpinia zerumbet and its main constituent 1,8-cineole in rats.' *Phytomedicine.* Dec v16(12):1151–5 http://www.sciencedirect.com/science/article/pii/S0944711309001226

77. Kehrl W., Sonnemann U., Dethlefsen U. (2004) 'Therapy for acute nonpurulent rhinosinusitis with cineole: results of a double-blind, randomized, placebo-controlled trial.' *Laryngoscope.* Apr v114(4):738–42 http://www.ncbi.nlm.nih.gov/pubmed/15064633

78. Tesche S. et al. (2008) 'The value of herbal medicines in the treatment of acute non-purulent rhinosinusitis. 'Results of a double-blind, randomised, controlled trial.' *Eur Arch Otorhinolaryngol.* Nov v265(11):1355–9 http://www.ncbi.nlm.nih.gov/pubmed/18437408

79. Worth H., Schacher C., Dethlefsen U. (2009) 'Concomitant therapy

with Cineole (Eucalyptole) reduces exacerbations in COPD: a placebo-controlled double-blind trial.' *Respir Res.* v10(1):6

80. Astani A., Reichling J., Schnitzler P. (2010) 'Comparative study on the antiviral activity of selected monoterpenes derived from essential oils.' *Phytotherapy Research.* v24(5):673–9 http://www.ncbi.nlm.nih.gov/pmc/articles/PMC2720945/

81. Matthys H. et al. (2000) 'Efficacy and tolerability of myrtol standardized in acute bronchitis. A multi-centre, randomised, double-blind, placebo-controlled parallel group clinical trial vs. cefuroxime and ambroxol.' *Arzneimittelforschung.* Aug v50(8):700–11 http://www.ncbi.nlm.nih.gov/pubmed/10994153

82. Meister R. et al. (1999) 'Efficacy and tolerability of myrtol standardized in long-term treatment of chronic bronchitis. A double-blind, placebo-controlled study. Study Group Investigators.' *Arzneimittelforschung.* Apr v49(4):351–8 https://www.researchgate.net/publication/12962202_Efficacy_and_tolerability_of_myrtol_standardized_in_long-term_treatment_of_chronic_bronchitis_A_double-blind_placebo-controlled_study_Study_Group_Investigators

83. Saito Y. et al. (2004) 'Effects of a novel gaseous antioxidative system containing a rosemary extract on the oxidation induced by nitrogen dioxide and ultraviolet radiation.' *Biosci Biotechnol Biochem.* Apr v68(4):781–6 http://www.ncbi.nlm.nih.gov/pubmed/15118303

84. Nasel C. et al. (1994) 'Functional imaging of effects of fragrances on the human brain after prolonged inhalation.' *Chem Senses.* Aug v19(4):359–64 http://www.ncbi.nlm.nih.gov/pubmed/7812728

85. Wächtler B. et al. (2012) 'Candida albicans-epithelial interactions: dissecting the roles of active penetration, induced endocytosis and host factors on the infection process.' PLOS One. 7(5) http://journals.plos.org/plosone/article?id=10.1371/journal.pone.0036952

86. Fan D. et al. (2015) 'Activation of HIF-1α and LL-37 by commensal bacteria inhibits Candida albicans colonization.' *Nature Medicine.* v21:808–14 http://www.nature.com/nm/journal/v21/n7/full/nm.3871.html

87. Souza C. L. et al. (2015) 'Commitment of human pluripotent stem cells to a neural lineage is induced by the pro-estrogenic flavonoid apigenin.' *Advances in Regenerative Biology.* v2 http://www.regenerativebiology.net/index.php/arb/article/view/29244

88. Hamidpour M. et al. (2014) 'Chemistry, pharmacology, and medicinal property of sage (Salvia) to prevent and cure illnesses such as obesity, diabetes, depression, dementia, lupus, autism, heart disease, and cancer.' *J Tradit Complement Med.* Apr–Jun; v4(2):82–8. http://www.ncbi.nlm.nih.gov/pubmed/24860730

89. Diego M. A. et al. (1998) 'Aromatherapy positively affects mood, EEG patterns of alertness and math computations.' *Int. J Neurosci.*

v96(3–4):217–24   http://www.tandfonline.com/doi/abs/10.3109/00207459808986469

90. Sayorwan W. (2012) 'The effects of lavender oil inhalation on emotional states, autonomic nervous system and brain electrical activity.' *J Med Assoc Thai.* Apr v95(4):598–606 http://www.ncbi.nlm.nih.gov/pubmed/22612017

91. Chaput J. P., Tremblay A. (2012) 'Adequate sleep to improve the treatment of obesity.' *CMAJ.* v184(18):1975–6. http://www.ncbi.nlm.nih.gov/pmc/articles/PMC3519150/

92. Deane J. (2010) 'Compulsive overeating & binge eating disorder, National Centre for Eating Disorders.' http://eating-disorders.org.uk/information/compulsive-overeating-binge-eating-disorder/

93. Woelk H., Schläfke S. (2010) 'A multi-center, double-blind, randomised study of the Lavender oil preparation Silexan in comparison to Lorazepam for generalized anxiety disorder.' *Phytomedicine.* Feb v17(2):94–9. http://www.ncbi.nlm.nih.gov/pubmed/19962288/

94. Borek C. (2006) 'Garlic reduces dementia and heart-disease risk.' *J Nutr.* Mar v136(3): 810S–12S http://jn.nutrition.org/content/136/3/810S.full

95. Borek C. (2001) 'Antioxidant health effects of aged garlic extract.' *J Nutr.* Mar v131(3): 1010S–1015S http://jn.nutrition.org/content/131/3/1010S.full

96. Mathew B. C., Biju R. S. (2008) 'Neuroprotective effects of garlic: a review.' *Libyan J Med.* v3(1): 23–33. http://www.ncbi.nlm.nih.gov/pmc/articles/PMC3074326/

97. Elkins G., Rajab M. H., Marcus J. (2005) 'Complementary and alternative medicine use by psychiatric inpatients.' *Psychological Reports.* v96(1):163–6 https://www.researchgate.net/publication/7910933_Complementary_and_alternative_medicine_use_by_psychiatric_inpatients

98. Lee M. S. et al. (2011) 'Reduction of body weight by dietary garlic is associated with an increase in uncoupling protein mRNA expression and activation of AMP-activated protein kinase in diet-induced obese mice.' *J Nutr.* Nov v141(11):1947–53. http://www.ncbi.nlm.nih.gov/pubmed/21918057

99. Banerjee S. K., Maulik S. K. (2002) 'Effect of garlic on cardiovascular disorders: a review.' *Nutrition Journal.* v1(4) http://nutritionj.biomedcentral.com/articles/10.1186/1475-2891-1-4

100. Ali B. H. et al. (2008) 'Some phytochemical, pharmacological and toxicological properties of ginger (Zingiber officinale Roscoe): a review of recent research.' *Food Chem Toxicol.* Feb v46(2):409–20. http://www.ncbi.nlm.nih.gov/pubmed/17950516

101. Masuda Y. et al. (2004) 'Antioxidant properties of gingerol related compounds from ginger.' *Biofactors.* v21(1–4):293–6. http://www.ncbi.nlm.nih.gov/pubmed/15630214

102. Ghayur M. N. et al. (2008) 'Muscarinic, Ca(++) antagonist and specific butyrylcholinesterase inhibitory activity of dried ginger extract might explain its use in dementia.' *J Pharm Pharmacol.* Oct v60(10):1375–83. http://www.ncbi.nlm.nih.gov/pubmed/18812031

103. Saenghong N. et al. (2011) 'Zingiber officinale improves cognitive function of the middle-aged healthy women.' *Evid Based Complement Alternat Med.* v2012: 383062. http://www.ncbi.nlm.nih.gov/pmc/articles/PMC3253463/

104. Zeng G. F. et al. (2013) 'Protective effects of ginger root extract on Alzheimer disease-induced behavioral dysfunction in rats.' *Rejuvenation Res.* Apr v16(2):124–33. http://www.ncbi.nlm.nih.gov/pubmed/23374025

105. Waggas A. M. (2009) 'Neuroprotective evaluation of extract of ginger (Zingiber officinale) root in monosodium glutamate-induced toxicity in different brain areas male albino rats.' *Pak J Biol Sci.* Feb v12(3):201–12. http://science.naturalnews.com/2009/1230801_Neuroprotective_evaluation_of_extract_of_ginger_Zingiber_officinale_root_in.html

106. Li Y. et al. (2012) 'Preventive and protective properties of zingiber officinale (ginger) in diabetes mellitus, diabetic complications, and associated lipid and other metabolic disorders: a brief review.' *Evid Based Complement Alternat Med.* v2012 http://www.ncbi.nlm.nih.gov/pubmed/23243452

107. Aggarwal B. B. et al. (2007) 'Curcumin: the Indian solid gold.' *Adv Exp Med Biol.* v595:1–75. https://www.researchgate.net/publication/6268357_Curcumin_the_Indian_solid_gold_Adv_Exp_Med_Biol

108. Ejaz A. et al. (2009) 'Curcumin inhibits adipogenesis in 3T3-L1 adipocytes and angiogenesis and obesity in C57/BL mice.' *J Nutr.* May v139(5):919–25 http://www.ncbi.nlm.nih.gov/pubmed/19297423

109. Sanmukhani J. et al. (2014) 'Efficacy and safety of curcumin in major depressive disorder: a randomized controlled trial.' *Phytother Res.* Apr v28(4):579–85 http://www.ncbi.nlm.nih.gov/pubmed/23832433/

110. Kulkarni S. K., Dhir A. (2010) 'An overview of curcumin in neurological disorders.' indian *J Pharm Sci.* Mar–Apr v72(2):149–54 http://www.ncbi.nlm.nih.gov/pubmed/20838516

111. Mishra S., Palanivelu K. (2008) 'The effect of curcumin (turmeric) on Alzheimer's disease: an overview.' *Ann Indian Acad Neurol.* Jan–Mar v11(1):13–19. http://www.ncbi.nlm.nih.gov/pmc/articles/PMC2781139/#!po=39.4737

Chapter 10: Supporting Your Success

1. Baldwin A. L. (2011) 'Reiki, the Scientific Evidence.' pp. 29–31. https://reikiwitholivia.files.wordpress.com/2012/12/reikiscientificevidence.pdf

2. Baldwin A. L., Schwartz G. E. (2006) 'Personal interaction with a

reiki practitioner decreases noise-induced microvascular damage in an animal model.' *J Altern Complement Med* Jan–Feb v12(1):15–22, 2006. http://www.ncbi.nlm.nih.gov/pubmed/16494564

3. Baldwin A. L., Wagers C., Schwartz G. E. (2008) 'Reiki improves heart rate homeostasis in laboratory rats.' *J Altern Complement Med.* May v14(4):417–22. http://www.ncbi.nlm.nih.gov/pubmed/18435597

4. Diaz-Rodriguez L. et al. (2011) 'Immediate effects of reiki on heart rate variability, cortisol levels, and body temperature in health care professionals with burnout.' *Biol Res Nurs.* Oct v13(4): 376–82 http://www.ncbi.nlm.nih.gov/pubmed/21821642

5. Dressin L. J., Singg S. (1998) 'Effects of reiki on pain and selected affective and personality variables of chronically ill patients.' *Subtle Energies and Energy Medicine,* v9(1):53–82. http://www.reiki.it/sites/default/files/Effects_of%20_Reiki%20_on%20_pain.pdf

6. Friedman R. S. C. et al. (2010) 'Effects of reiki on autonomic activity early after acute coronary syndrome.' *J Am Col Cardiol.* v56: 995–6. http://reikiinmedicine.org/pdf/jacc.pdf

7. Shore A. G. (2004) 'Long term effects of energetic healing on symptoms of psychological depression and self-perceived stress.' *Altern Ther Health Med.* May–Jun v10(3):42–8. http://www.ncbi.nlm.nih.gov/pubmed/15154152

8. Vitale A. T., O'Conner P. C. (2006) 'The effect of reiki on pain and anxiety in women with abdominal hysterectomies.' *Holistic Nursing Practice.* v20(6):263–72. https://www.researchgate.net/publication/6698910_The_effect_of_Reiki_on_pain_and_anxiety_in_women_with_abdominal_hysterectomies_A_quasi-experimental_pilot_study

9. Weze C. et al. (2005) 'Evaluation of healing by gentle touch.' *Public Health.* v119(1):3–10. http://www.publichealthjrnl.com/article/S0033-3506(04)00077-0/abstract?cc=y=

10. Alandydy P., Alandydy K. (1999) 'Using reiki to support surgical patients.' *J Nur Care Qual.* Apr v13(4):89–91. https://www.researchgate.net/publication/12967514_Using_Reiki_To_Support_Surgical_Patients

11. Brewitt B., Vittetoe T., Hartwell B. (1997) 'The efficacy of reiki hands-on healing: improvements in spleen and nervous system function as quantified by electrodermal screening.' *Alternative Therapies.* v3(4):89

12. Mansour A. et al. (1999) 'A study to test the effectiveness of placebo reiki standardization procedures developed for a planned reiki efficacy study.' *J Altern Complement Med.* Apr v5(2):153–64. http://www.ncbi.nlm.nih.gov/pubmed/10328637

13. American Psychological Association website (2012) 'The Impact of Stress.' Retrieved from: http://www.apa.org/news/press/releases/stress/2012/impact.aspx?item=2

14. Health and Safety Executive website (2012) 'Stress and Psychological Disorders.' http://www.hse.gov.uk/statistics/index.htm

15. Halliwell E. (2010) 'The Mindfulness Report.' http://www.livingmindfully.co.uk/downloads/Mindfulness_Report.pdf

16. Benson H., Beary J. F., Carol M. P. (1974) 'The relaxation response.' *Psychiatry.* v37:37–45

17. Goldin P., Gross J. (2010) 'Effects of mindfulness-based stress reduction (MBSR) on emotion regulation in social anxiety disorder.' *Emotion.* Feb v10(1): 83–91. http://www.ncbi.nlm.nih.gov/pubmed/20141305

18. Hölzel B. et al. (2011) 'Mindfulness practice leads to increases in regional brain gray matter density.' *Psychiatry Res.* Jan v191(1):36–43. http://www.ncbi.nlm.nih.gov/pmc/articles/PMC3004979/

19. Mackenzie C. R., Poulin P. A., Seidman-Carlson R. (2006) 'A brief mindfulness-based stress reduction intervention for nurses and nurse aides.' *Applied Nursing Research.* May v19(2):105–9 http://www.appliednursingresearch.org/article/S0897-1897(06)00008-5/abstract?cc=y=

20. Ostafin B. D., Kassman K. T. (2012) 'Stepping out of history: mindfulness improves insight problem solving.' *Conscious Cogn.* Jun v21(2):1031–6. http://www.ncbi.nlm.nih.gov/pubmed/22483682

21. Colzato L. S., Ozturk A., Hommel B. (2012) 'Meditate to create: the impact of focused-attention and open-monitoring training on convergent and divergent thinking.' *Front. Psychology.* Apr v3(1):116. https://www.researchgate.net/publication/224821975_Meditate_to_Create_The_Impact_of_Focused-Attention_and_Open-Monitoring_Training_on_Convergent_and_Divergent_Thinking

22. Greenberg J., Reiner K., Meiran N. (2012) '"Mind the trap": mindfulness practice reduces cognitive rigidity.' PLOS One. May v7(5). http://www.ncbi.nlm.nih.gov/pmc/articles/PMC3352909/

23. Moffitt T. et al. (2011) 'From the cover: a gradient of childhood self-control predicts health, wealth, and public safety.' *Proc Natl Acad Sci.* Feb v108(7):2693–8. http://www.ncbi.nlm.nih.gov/pmc/articles/PMC3041102/

24. Mischel W., Shoda Y., Peake P. K. (1988) 'The nature of adolescent competencies predicted by preschool delay of gratification.' *J Pers Soc Psychol.* Apr v54(4):687–96. http://www.ncbi.nlm.nih.gov/pubmed/3367285

25. Duckworth A. L., Seligman M. E. P. (2005) 'Self-discipline outdoes IQ in predicting academic performance of adolescents.' *Psychological Science.* Dec v16(12):939–44. http://pss.sagepub.com/content/16/12/939.short

26. Dietz P. et al. (2013) 'Randomized response estimates for the 12-month prevalence of cognitive-enhancing drug use in university students.' *Pharmacotherapy: The Journal of Human Pharmacology and Drug Therapy.* Jan v33(1):44–50. http://onlinelibrary.wiley.com/doi/10.1002/phar.1166/abstract

27. Levy D. et al. (2012) 'The Effects of Mindfulness Meditation Training on Multitasking in a High-Stress Information Environment.' Proceedings of Graphics Interface Conference pp. 45–52. https://faculty.washington.edu/wobbrock/pubs/gi-12.02.pdf

28. MacLean K. A. et al. (2010) 'Intensive meditation training improves perceptual discrimination and sustained attention.' *Psychol Sci.* Jun v21(6):829–39. http://www.ncbi.nlm.nih.gov/pmc/articles/PMC3132583

29. Jha A. P. et al. (2010) 'Examining the protective effects of mindfulness training on working memory capacity and affective experience.' *Emotion.* Feb v10(1):54–64. http://www.ncbi.nlm.nih.gov/pubmed/20141302

30. Zeidan F. et al. (2010) 'Mindfulness meditation improves cognition: Evidence of brief mental training.' *Conscious Cogn.* Jun v19(2):597–605. http://www.ncbi.nlm.nih.gov/pubmed/20363650

31. Tang Y. et al. (2010) 'Short-term meditation induces white matter changes in the anterior cingulate.' *Proc Natl Acad Sci USA.* Aug v107(35):15649–52. http://www.ncbi.nlm.nih.gov/pmc/articles/PMC2932577

32. Michael T., Zetsche U., Margraf J. (2007) 'Epidemiology of anxiety disorders.' *Psychiatry.* Apr v6(4):136–42. http://www.sciencedirect.com/science/article/pii/S1476179307000237

33. Sedlmeier P. et al. (2012) 'The psychological effects of meditation: a meta-analysis.' *Psychological Bulletin.* v138(6):1139–71. https://www.thehartcenter.com//wp-content/uploads/2011/11/Meditation-Metta-Analysis-American-Psychologist-.pdf

34. Kabat-Zinn J. et al. (1992) 'Effectiveness of a meditation-based stress reduction program in the treatment of anxiety disorders.' *Am J Psychiatry.* Jul v149(7):936–43. http://www.ncbi.nlm.nih.gov/pubmed/1609875

35. Hofmann S. G. et al. (2010) 'The effect of mindfulness-based therapy on anxiety and depression: a meta-analytic review.' *J Consult Clin Psychol.* Apr v78(2):169–83. http://www.ncbi.nlm.nih.gov/pubmed/20350028

36. Goldin P. R., Gross J. J. (2010) 'Effects of mindfulness-based stress reduction (MBSR) on emotion regulation in social anxiety disorder.' *Emotion.* Feb v10(1):83–91. http://www.ncbi.nlm.nih.gov/pubmed/20141305

37. Hölzel B. K. et al. (2009) 'Stress reduction correlates with structural changes in the amygdala.' *Soc Cogn Affect Neurosci.* Mar v5(1):11–17. http://www.ncbi.nlm.nih.gov/pmc/articles/PMC2840837/

Chapter 11: The Future – You Can Do It!

1. 'Prescription drugs: 7 out of 10 Americans take at least one, study finds (2015).' *Huffington Post* http://www.huffingtonpost.com/2013/06/19/prescription-drugs-prevalence-americans_n_3466801.html